A 100% Vegetarian Diet

Staying Healthy through Vegetarian Foods

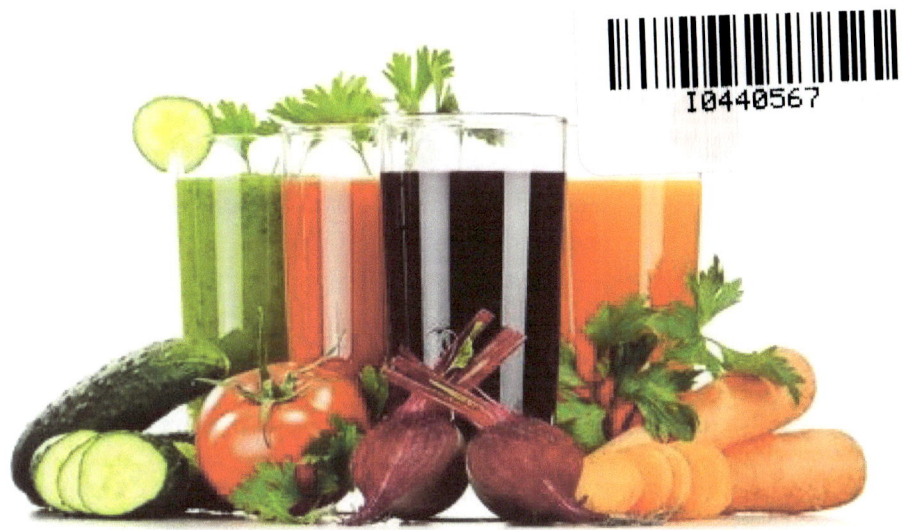

I0440567

Dueep Jyot Singh

Healthy Living Series

Mendon Cottage Books

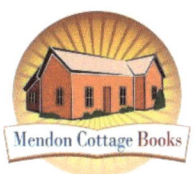

JD-Biz Publishing

Download Free Books!

http://MendonCottageBooks.com

All Rights Reserved.

No part of this publication may be reproduced in any form or by any means, including scanning, photocopying, or otherwise without prior written permission from JD-Biz Corp Copyright © 2015

All Images Licensed by Fotolia and 123RF.

Disclaimer

The information is this book is provided for informational purposes only. It is not intended to be used and medical advice or a substitute for proper medical treatment by a qualified health care provider. The information is believed to be accurate as presented based on research by the author.

The contents have not been evaluated by the U.S. Food and Drug Administration or any other Government or Health Organization and the contents in this book are not to be used to treat cure or prevent disease.

The author or publisher is not responsible for the use or safety of any diet, procedure or treatment mentioned in this book. The author or publisher is not responsible for errors or omissions that may exist.

Warning

The Book is for informational purposes only and before taking on any diet, treatment or medical procedure, it is recommended to consult with your primary health care provider.

Our books are available at

1. Amazon.com
2. Barnes and Noble
3. Itunes
4. Kobo
5. Smashwords
6. Google Play Books

Table of Contents

Introduction

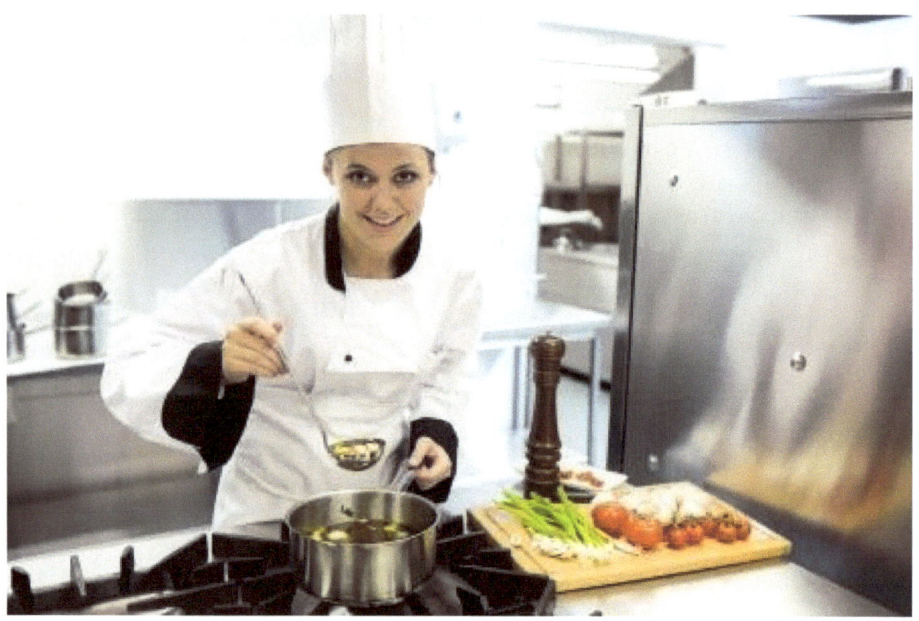

For centuries people have been very particular about the things they eat. What should be eaten, what should not be eaten, what should be eaten within its spanned season, and other factors related to food, are a part and parcel of our daily lives.

This book is going to give you plenty of information about how a vegetarian diet can keep you healthy and long-lived, along with a number of recipes, which you can incorporate into your lifestyle right now. And for all those people who cannot do without their pizzas, one of the recipes is going to include a magnificent traditional pizza recipe.

Down the ages, people have known that they are some essential nutrients, which are available only in the bounty of nature, and which cannot be obtained by any other resource. These are vitamins, proteins, carbohydrates, fats, minerals, and other essential nutrients, which are necessary to keep you healthy and strong.

The main duty of food is to give you strength through natural nourishment, and build the tissue up in a healthy fashion. Food also gives you warmth, energy, and allows the life systems to work properly. Apart from that, food builds up your immune system, and protects you from a number of ailments.

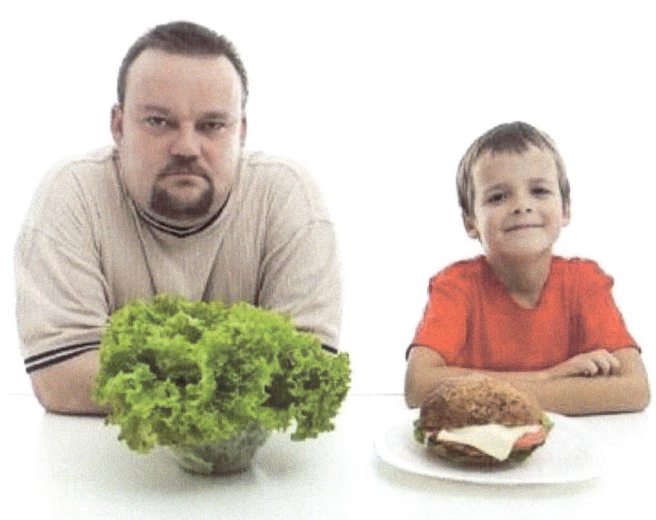

This book is going to give you plenty of information on how a vegetarian diet can help you keep healthy. Thanks to the nourishment content, these greens, vegetables and fruit, which come under a vegetarian diet are going to help keep you strong throughout your lifetime.

The word vegetarian does not come from vegetables, as you may assume, but from the Latin word "vegetus" which stands for "active" or "full of energy". It describes a diet, where a person refrains from a diet consisting of meat and instead eats fruit, nuts, seeds, and even eggs in his diet.

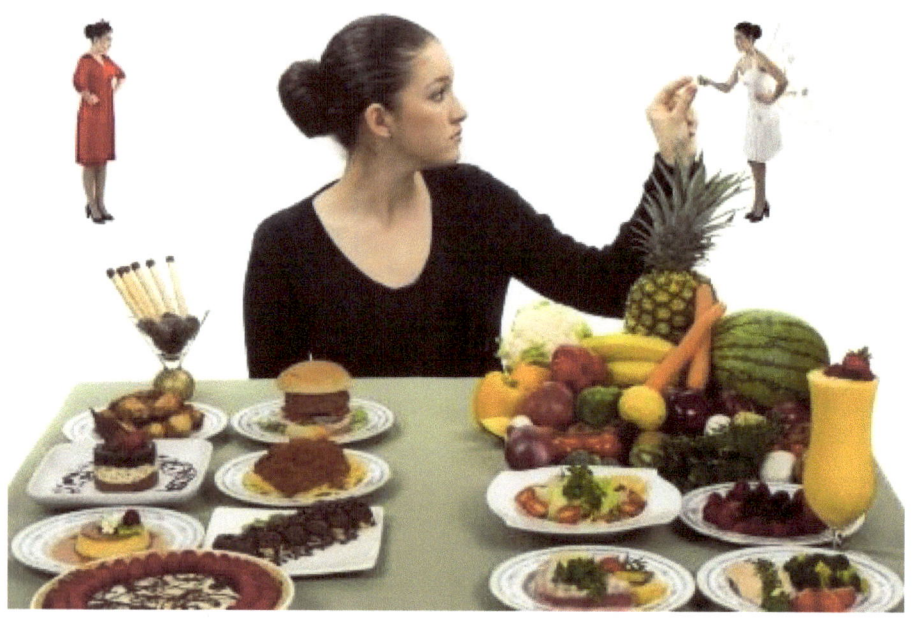

In 1961, research was done, why many Americans suffered from cancer of the stomach or cancer of the colon. It was found that their diet was responsible for the prevalence of these ailments. That is why, in 1970, Americans decided to change their eating habits and lifestyles drastically. They began to look towards a vegetarian diet and began to incorporate it into their own daily diet and lifestyle.

Europe followed and that is the reason why, today a vegetarian diet is considered to be one of the most healthy diets available to mankind as it was available to mankind millenniums ago.

Ancient holy books talked about a diet, which was "pure" and which meant eating the fruit of the earth in the shape of vegetables, fruits, nuts, roots, bark, and other natural gifts of the Gods, off trees, herbs, shrubs, and vines.

In fact, they believed that as long as the food was eaten naturally, in its original form without being tampered – by which we mean steaming, roasting, broiling, frying, baking – one would derive the most benefit out of it. Naturally, no one could eat his meat raw. It had to be cooked in order to be digestible. That is why it was not eaten by the ancients very often.

If you find yourself suffering from a large number of trivial ailments, which means that your immune system is not so strong, try eating 100% vegetarian diet. This is going to include raw vegetables, green vegetables, salads, and fruit. You are going to drink milk, or fresh fruit juice.

I remember going to my cousin's wedding where his cousin – from his mother's side – who was to be married within the fortnight was also a guest. Her skin was glowing, she looked marvelous, and everyone envied her future bridegroom! This was the young girl with teenage acne, puppy fat, and a number of other problems related to overeating because she just could not be stopped when confronted with butter, ham, hamburgers, and anything else of which you could think.

She told me that when the boy's family came to ask for her hand, she was made up so heavily that she looked absolutely stunning. The wedding was fixed for six months later. Her father, being a go getting Colonel, acted immediately.

She was immediately put in the hands of a naturopathy Hermitage – of which they are plenty in our country, where you go back two millenniums, eating, drinking, and working like the people of that time, and come out very youthful looking, completely healthy, and lovely to look at!

When Ginny came for our cousin's wedding, she had been drinking fresh fruit juice, in that Hermitage, for the past one month, until she told us that she would never want to drink it ever again. Apart from that, she was given fruit, nuts, vegetables, green vegetables, and other vegetarian food, cooked deliciously in such a manner that she never even felt the craving for a raw juicy steak!

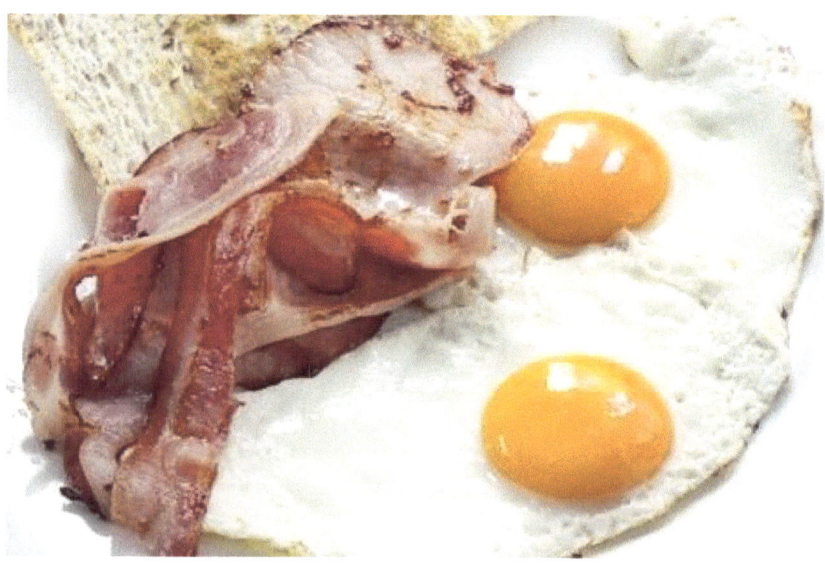

As a child, I could not do without a bacon and eggs breakfast, with plenty of hot buttered toast and jam, followed by a glass of hot milk before I went to school, but as an adult, on a vegetarian diet, I have to say goodbye to it reluctantly…

According to Socrates, the food that you eat is what keeps you healthy, and what keeps you free of diseases. But then Socrates was definitely not too much of a meat eater, because at that time meat, lamb, fish, and other non-vegetarian food items could be afforded by only those people who were prosperous. He as a philosopher was definitely not prosperous.

Incidentally, this was the time when Roman cooking was at its Zenith. The best parts of the meat went to the people who were prosperous; the priests and the rich aristocrats. The common folk had to do with the bones, the entrails, the hooves, and other discarded parts of the animal.

This is when ingenuity came into play. They used herbs, spices, and other ingredients like milk, seeds, nuts, and honey to make even the most originally unappetizing looking piece of offal into a dish fit for a Caesar.

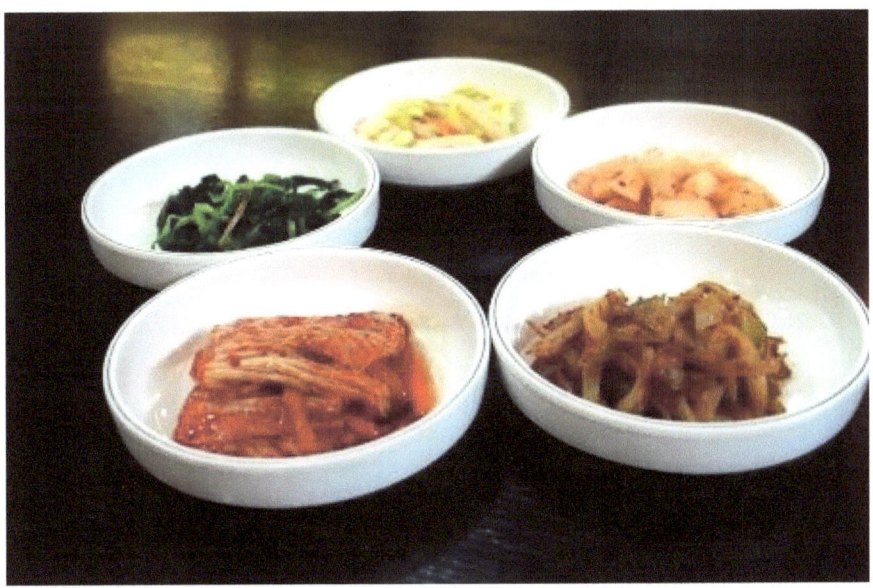

These are traditional vegetable and herb in vinegar accompaniments to meals coming down from that particular time.

However, they made sure that their diets were full of lots of vegetable and fruit matter. Because many times, they could not even get that offal. So this is the reason why they were strong, healthy, and managed to bring up their families on fruit, green vegetables, roots, nuts, herbs and spices along with milk, if they could get it.

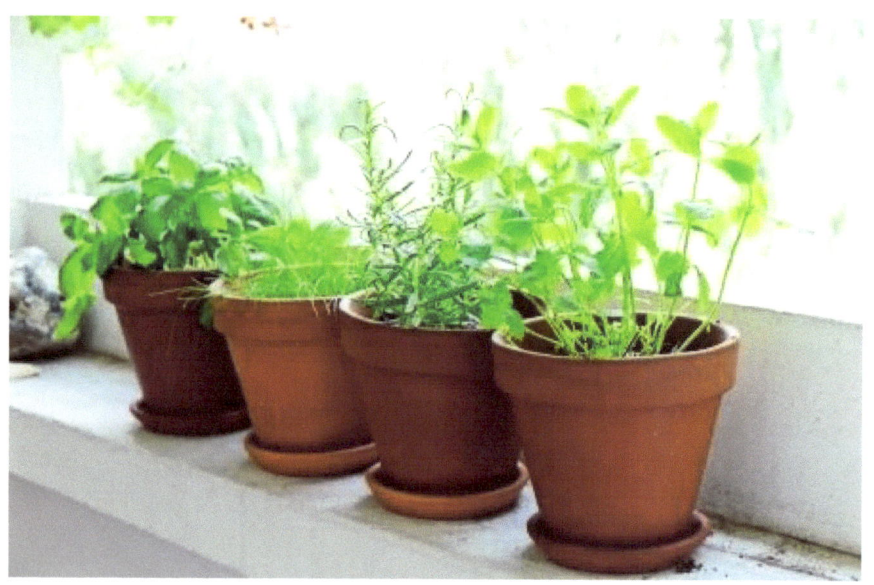

Herbs added to your daily diet are going to make your food much more palatable.

So what happens if you do not have important vitamins and nutrients in your meal? A vitamin C deficiency was one of the banes of sailors down the centuries, and in one of the books written by a Viking ship's captain more than 2000 years ago, he advises the sailors when they reach one particular island to embark there, and eat the grasses. Also, he said that the fruit and the vegetables in that particular island would help get rid of all the ailments incurred during their long journey, and they would be ready to go on their return trip, healthy and strong.

These fruit, vegetables, and grasses definitely contain plenty of vitamins C and other minerals. This meant that the scurvy incurred during the long journey, by eating just ship tack, hard biscuits, fish, and other preserved meat products and definitely no fruit and vegetables, was counteracted with this intake of minerals, vitamins, and other nutritious natural food elements.

The Importance of Vitamin C in Your Diet

So if you find yourself looking pale and anemic, with bleeding gums and loosened teeth, feel lethargic, feel pain in the body, it is a sign that you are suffering from a vitamin C deficiency. Start your intake of citrus fruit immediately, including lemons, oranges, and other citrus fruit. Incidentally, a vitamin C deficiency is going to cause halitosis and bad breath.

This is the reason why in ancient times, people suffering from bad breath were told to drink plenty of lemon juice, gargle with lemon and saltwater and brush their teeth with powdered salt and lemon peel. This kept their gums healthy, and prevented their teeth from rotting and falling out.

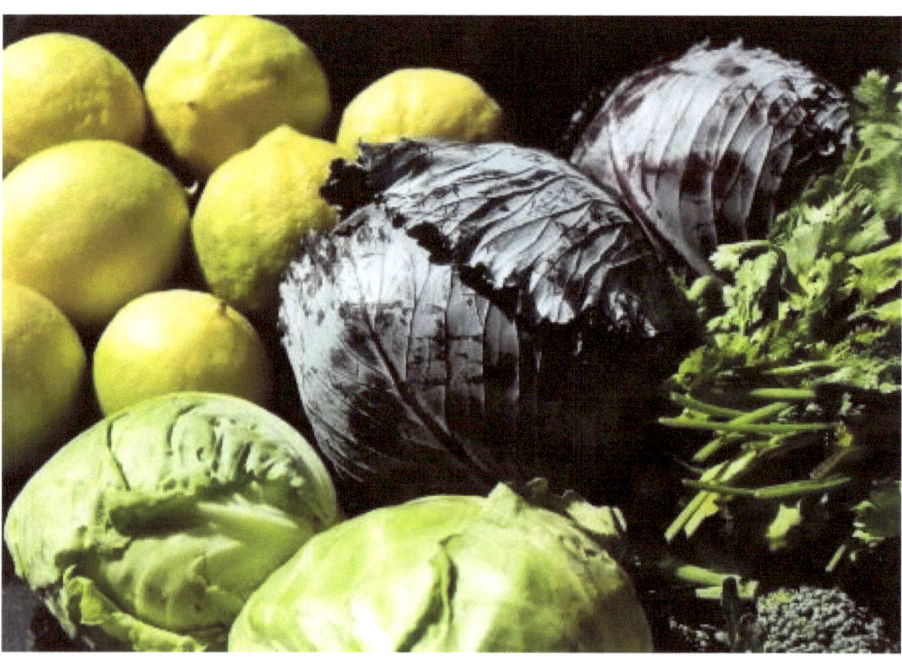

A vitamin C deficiency can also have an adverse effect on your bones, tissues, and muscles. The wounds are not going to heal properly and in time. And even a small cut could cause extensive bleeding. Also, just one little slip and you may find all your bones breaking because they have grown so brittle.

Incidentally, stop your vitamin C intake, and see the effect it is going to have upon your temper. You may find yourself losing your temper, even more often! That is because you feel weak, lethargic, and find that you cannot concentrate properly. By the way, you need plenty of vitamin C in your diet, if you want to keep your heart strong and healthy.

Also, apart from weakness, you are going to find yourself more prone to infections because your immune system is all shot to pieces. This includes chest problems, including cold, pneumonia, cough, and other nose and throat ailments.

Vitamin C keeps your stomach, digestive system, and liver healthy. It helps your body to grow, allows you to put on weight naturally, makes you feel a healthy hunger, and supports the renewed growth of red blood corpuscles.

In its natural form, you are going to find it in oranges, lemons, limes, and other citric fruit, which are juicy. In vegetables, you are going to find vitamin C in cabbages, lettuces, young cauliflowers, small baby carrots, tomatoes, onions, coriander, radishes, beetroots, spinach, pineapples, gooseberries, pears, and guavas.

If you find a place where you can get dried gooseberries powder, or you can dry gooseberries yourself, under the shade, outside, in one corner of your porch, allow them to dry out completely. It is going to take 3 to 4 days for you to do this.

Now collect these dried gooseberries, and grind them finely. Every day, you are going to have half a teaspoonful of this powder with one teaspoonful of honey, in the morning, for the next four months.

I said four months, because I intend to cure you of your chronic ailments and that is about the time taken for curing them. Teensy weensy ailments will have diminished, long before then.

This is going to help cure chronic insomnia, strengthen your powers of concentration, strengthen your heart, darken your hair, get rid of chronic headaches. You can also dry the powder off and make them into pellets. Eat six small pellets, three times a day, to find the power of the gooseberry making you young, strong, and healthy.

Green vegetables are normally be eaten without cooking. You can also take them in juice form, drunk immediately after juicing. This is extremely good for your longevity prospects.

Vitamin A

Vitamin A is excellent for eyesight. As a child, I suffered badly from shortsightedness and was half blind till the age of 22. My grandmother tried to get rid of the vitamin A deficiency by feeding me lots of fresh greens and salads, cabbages, coriander, green mint leaves, the young green leaves of radishes, fenugreek leaves, spinach, carrots, papayas, and of course, lots of homemade butter!

I never suffered from this deficiency, even though my eyes did not get well. They could not because I kept reading late into the darkness of the night with my covers drawn over me, and with the help of a torch! But she tried her best!

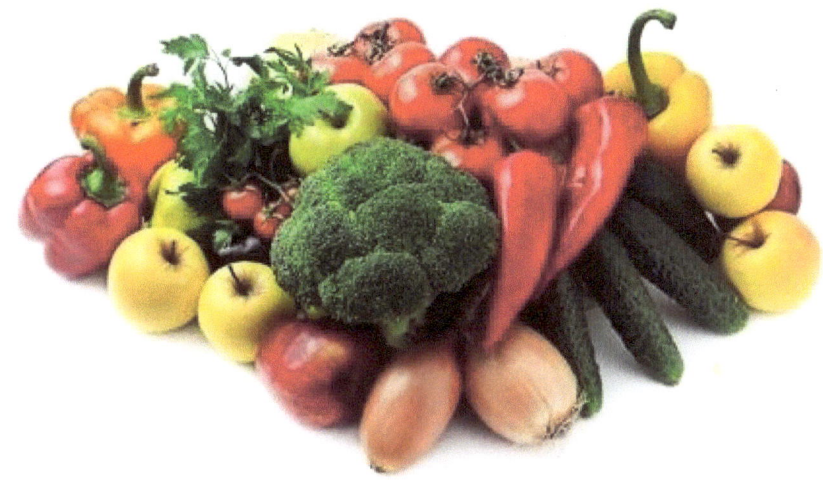

Nevertheless, thanks to these greens, I never suffered from night blindness. Also, my eyes shone with good health behind my horn rimmed frames,

One of the major benefits of this diet during childhood was that I would never suffered from stones as an adult. I do not. No stones in the gallbladder or in the kidney. So if you are suffering from any sort of uric acid build up, begin eating the vegetables and fruit, I mentioned above. If you can get homemade butter, so much the better!

All these vegetables have to be eaten raw. You can also make them into ground chutney, especially mint, coriander, and green radish leaves. Delicious!

They also delicious in juice form, especially spinach juice and green radish leaf juice mixed with carrots, mint, and coriander.

Continue drinking this mixture for about three months and see the change in your health, a visible change in your eyesight, and also a toxin free body.

Proteins

Many of us are in the impression that our protein intake can only be fulfilled by eating lots of meat, fish, and protein based food items. Surprisingly, while traveling, as a child, I found myself living in a state where traditionally, religiously, and culturally, they did not eat meat or eggs!

Oh my. Not eat meat at all? What on earth did they eat?

I soon found out that for millenniums, these people had fine-tuned a diet system, with lots of fruit, vegetables, milk products, mixed with delicious herbs, spices, and dry fruit. I still remember how tasty their meals were. Delicately flavored with spices, and the aroma of fresh homemade butter floating on the surface, these were mouthwatering and really delicious.

They got their proteins from beans. And a no meat diet did not prevent them at all from growing tall, slim, handsome, and very attractive looking. These proteinaceous amino acids out of which 23 were required by the body were supplied by grains, cereals, milk, and vegetables.

The traditional staple diet of rice, green vegetables, and lentils/beans, which has been a part and parcel of their culture for millenniums provided them with all the proteins necessary to keep them healthy and going strong.

Gaining Full Benefit of Vegetables and Fruit

How to Use Vegetables Effectively

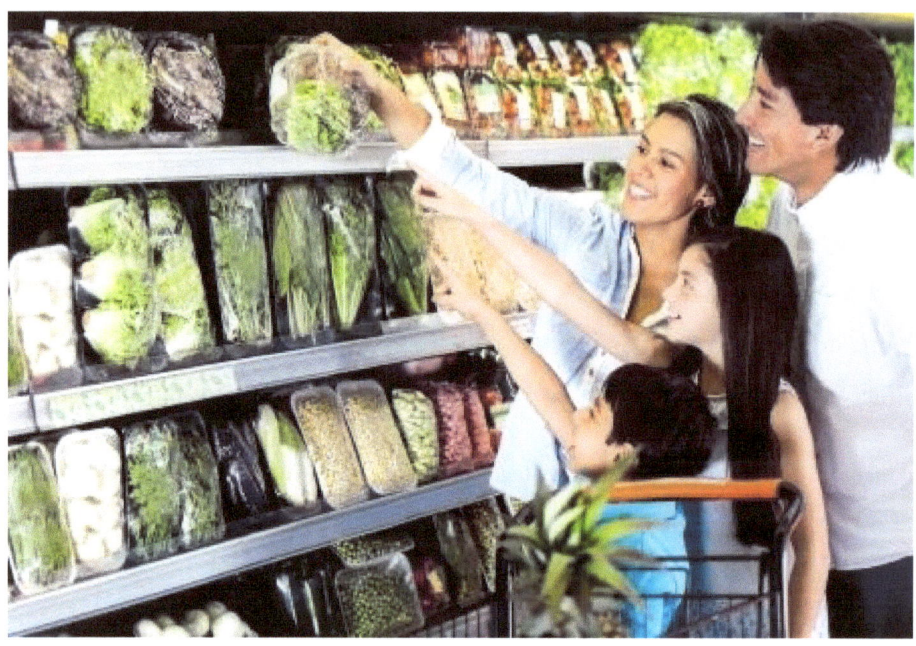

Most of us are so used to going into the vegetable section of our supermarket and picking up all the different packets there. According to us, they are fresh, because they have just been stocked in the shelves that morning. However, packaging causes many of these vegetables to grow stale with the passing of time.

If we are lucky enough to have a kitchen garden in which we are growing a large number of vegetables, we are going to have a really good supply of fresh, leafy, and green vegetables to add to our daily diet. These are going to take care of all the bio physiological functions of our body and make sure that it works in a proper and naturally healthy manner.

So when you are getting ready to select vegetables, make sure that they are fresh, green, leafy and full of fibers. They should not have any blemishes or marks, or fungal spots.

You cannot use any other food item or chemically manufactured supplement as a substitute for healthy, leafy, and fresh vegetables. Apart from imparting lots of variety and taste to your food, these vegetables help in the manufacture of digestive juices, speeding up your metabolism, and circulatory system, strengthening your immune system, rectifying your digestive system, and adding to your state of good health.

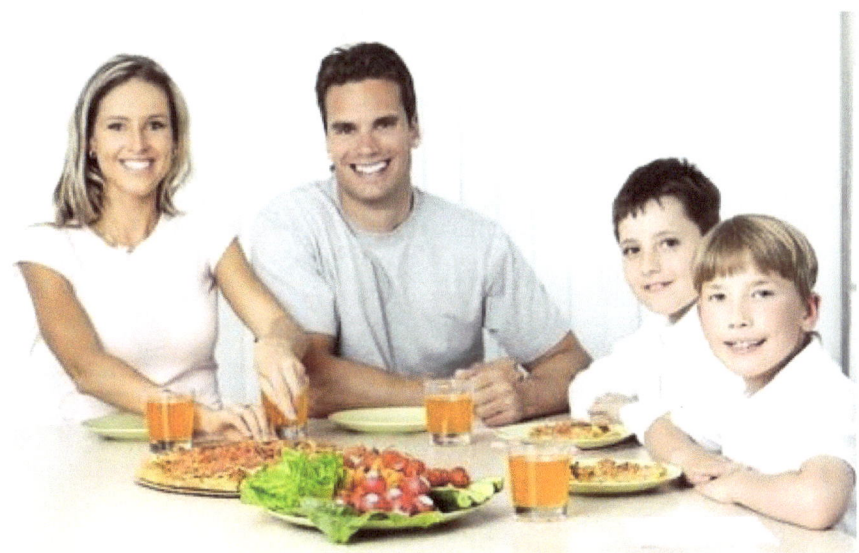

So here are some common sense and useful tips, which you need to implement whenever you go out to gather those green leafy vegetables.

If the leaves are very green and leafy, they are going to wilt faster, when compared to vegetables which are not leafy. That is why it is more sensible to use them right away, rather than wrapping them up in wet cloth and putting them in the fridge.

We have a weekly farmers market in our area every Friday. That is the time when the people in our neighborhood and beyond visit this large market and choose vegetables for the rest of the week. Tomatoes and potatoes can be preserved till next Friday, but spinach, cabbages, lettuce, and other green leafy vegetables are bought to be eaten within the next two days, in salads or cooked.

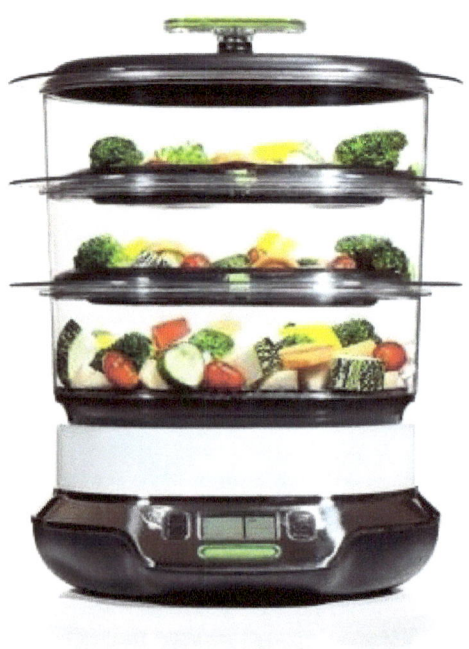

Steaming vegetables helps preserve the nutrient matter present in them, while making the food even tastier.

The best thing about this farmers market is that we do not have to bother about the middlemen. The prices are fixed early in the morning, and by night time, they are reduced to about 80% of the morning's price because the farmers do not want to take their vegetables back home in their tractors and trucks.

I was astonished to see a farmer dumping his stock of tomatoes on the road, a couple of months ago. One only has to blame the country's or state's government for this state of affairs, because there was no way in which the farmers in our State could send their excess glut of tomatoes to other States or even export them abroad. They did not have the infrastructure, nor the know-how. And this is the 21st-century!

So these vegetables were dumped on the road. And they rotted there, because the people of our State were too dignified to pick up free vegetables from off the streets.

What a pity, I told myself. A little bit of sense and application, and all these tomatoes could be turned by the family members of the farmers into local produce like sauces and chutneys. But one would rather dump vegetables on the road, then do something constructive and prosperous which entails a little bit of hard work.

So next time you get the vegetables of your choice, just wipe them with a clean cloth to get rid of the dust. You are going to wash them, only before you cook them. Continuous washing is going to get rid of all the essential nutrients below the surface of the skin.

Radish leaves, tomatoes, carrots, and beetroots should be eaten raw, as far as possible. The more you chew them, the more they are going to help aid in the digestion because when they are mixed up with the saliva, they become very powerful digestive agents.

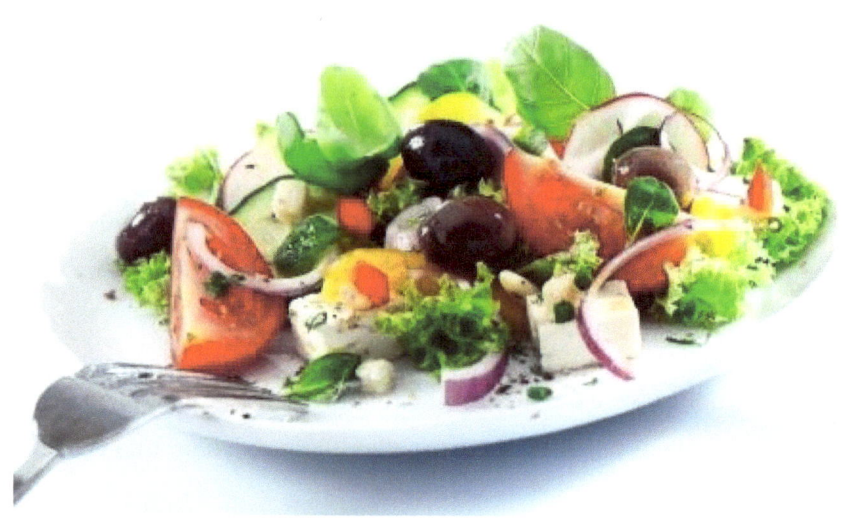

As kids, we were not encouraged to eat between meals, but our meals always had carrots and tomatoes and other green leafy vegetables as salads. These vegetables were freshly obtained from the garden, and fed to us within the hour. We were told to munch the carrots as often as we could, because that exercise would strengthen our teeth, gums, and jaws. It did! Much better than chewing gum and healthier.

Look at all the traditional cuisines, modern and ancient. Food is always served fresh, after it has been cooked with care. In ancient times, the members of the family were so hungry that they finished up every meal. At that time, the amount of food was also limited, and it was very rare that food would be left over for another helping at the next meal time.

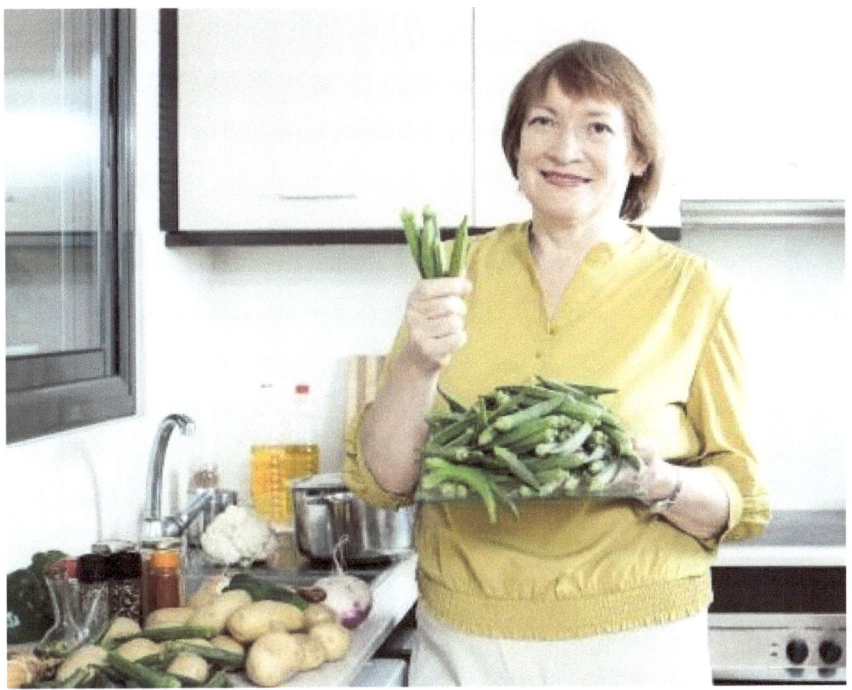

That is why everything was cooked fresh and fed fresh. But thanks to the preservative methods of the modern age, the lady of the house cooks just once in the morning, and the whole family is going to eat this food throughout the rest of the day. Some ladies cook just once a week, and put the food items away in the freezer to be defrosted when needed.

That is perhaps due to the fact that we are more bothered about expediency and time-saving than in eating freshly cooked food at the right time. So as far as possible, eat your fresh meal, within two – three hours and try not to put the leftovers in the fridge.

However, if it is necessary for you to preserve some green leafy vegetables, wrap them up in a wet paper – not a print paper – until it is airtight. You can also use airtight polythene bags. I have found a number of vegetable bags being sold by a large number of suppliers globally which are made up of a mixture of polythene, polyester and cloth. These are very sturdy and I have managed to keep vegetables in them for about four – five days, when I could not cook them right away.

http://www.amazon.com/flip-tumble-Reusable-Produce-Bags/dp/B002UXQ7QQ/ref=sr_1_2?ie=UTF8&qid=1443335251&sr=8-2&keywords=Vegetables+storage+mesh+bags

I found these rates very exorbitant, but you can always look for bargains now that you know what to look for, in your choice of polyester or cotton mesh bags.

Fruit Juice Cures

For all those people who are suffering from a weak digestion, they are going to find this condition much improved on a diet of fruit and vegetable juice in which water has been added. This is going to aid in the digestion of these juices.

Fruit should normally be eaten in the morning, on an empty stomach. This is going to benefit you even more, when you accompany it with fresh fruit juice.

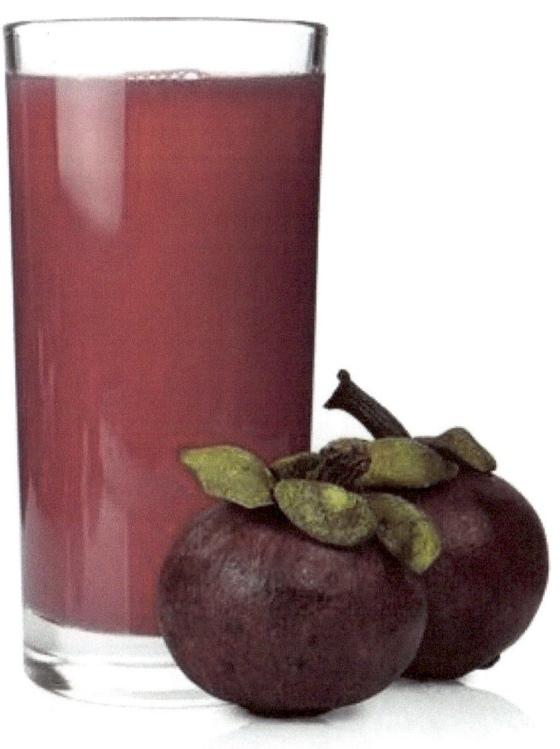

Fruit juices should always be drank fresh and raw. Curing yourselves through fruit juices is going to take a little while, because the body is going to have to accustom itself to this fresh, healthy product, when once it was used to toxins harming it.

It is going to take you a little while for you to cure yourself through fruit juices, but that is when patience is going to give you the best result. You can also use other supporting herbs and vegetables to help cure you faster.

Drink the juice, in the afternoon and in the morning. The amount you should drink in one day should be 16 ounces. You can mix seasonal vegetables, green vegetables, and even fruit to the mixture, according to your taste. Do not add sugar to this mixture. Many of us have the habit of doing that because we have got so used to drinking fruit juice concentrates with plenty of corn syrup in them, that it is going to take us a little while in order to get used to the taste of real honest to goodness fruit juice.

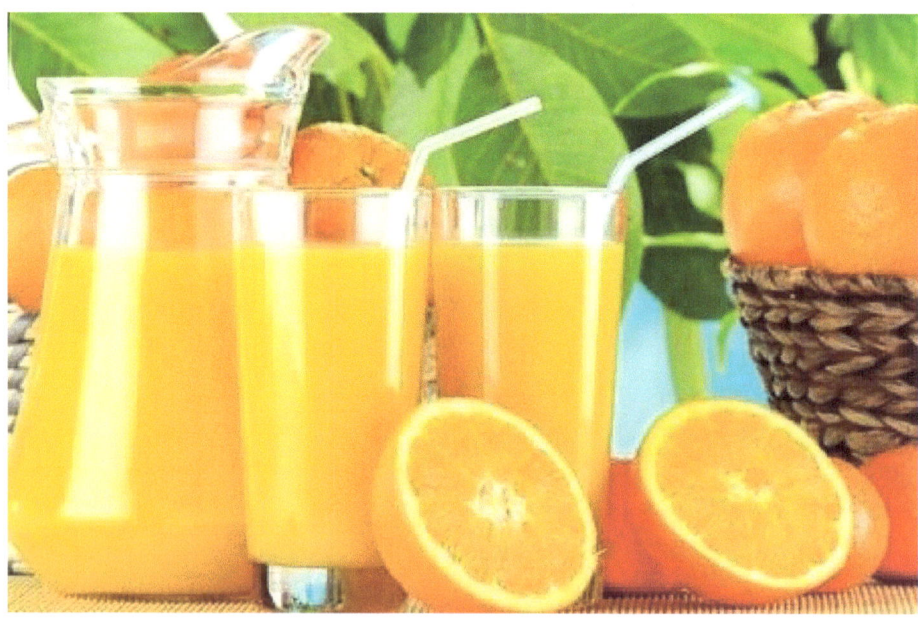

Fruit Peels

When we were at college, we used to play a really funny game. The moment an apple came into our hands, we would start at the very top and peel it very carefully, so that the peel did not break. After that, amidst howls of great cheers, the damsel peeling the apple would twirl it three times over her head and then allow it to fall over her right shoulder. The accompanying Greek chorus would immediately eye the shape of the fallen apple peel and see whether it fell into the shape of an alphabet or not.

Many times, it was wishful thinking, but many of these damsels "read" the first letter of their swains' names prophesied in the fallen apple peel. After that they had to eat that apple, saying his name, and there you are! Half an hour, every day of ladies crunching apples after having peeled them and twirled them and read their future marital bliss in them!

I found this game to be very psychologically interesting. Whoever thought this up made sure that that female ate an apple, good for her health – while chanting the name of a boy of the village/town/tribe. There would be someone somewhere ready to go and tell the boy's family that the girl was willing to accept an offer of marriage. And in those days, the marriage would take place.

Also, if the peel showed the shape of the first letter of a very eligible boy who was being courted by a number of girls in the village, the girl who spoke his name first would be considered to be his chosen mate as spoken by fate through an apple peel augur!

However, today it is much better to eat that apple unpeeled. Especially, fruit, which do not have a very hard outer covering should be eaten without peeling. That is because most of the nourishing elements in fruits and vegetables are under the surface of the peel. And you are throwing them away or feeding them to the livestock, or putting them on the compost heap!

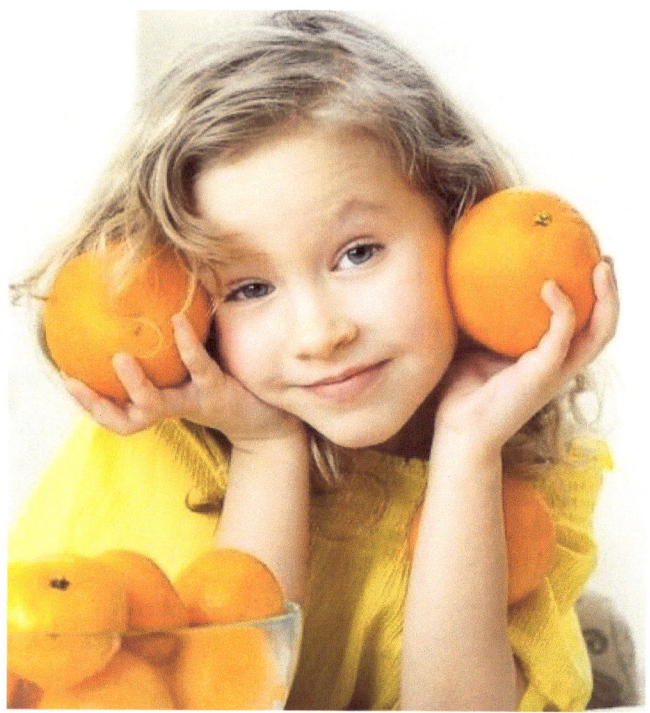

Besides, this roughage is excellent to keep your system healthy, as fiber. You are not going to suffer from constipation, if you keep eating apples unpeeled. This reminds me of a journey, I took in an open-air bus with the passenger sitting next to me with her brown paper bag full of oranges, bought from a street vendor.

She immediately took out one orange, and took a huge hefty bite of it, chomping up the peel too, in her enjoyment of her breakfast. I did not say anything about washing the fruit before eating it, because first of all, she was a stranger and I was a visitor to her land, and nobody talks in England, without being introduced first, but if she wanted to poison herself with non-organic fruit spray, that was her prerogative.

Nevertheless, in England, do as the Britans do, so I went to the next fruit vendor I saw, bought some oranges, washed them then and there and then spent the rest of the day, chomping – without peeling them – merrily away, riding on an open – air bus.

Incidentally, I got some – would-you-see-that – looks from other tourists, who are more used to eating their oranges, peeled. They were under the impression that people of my country eat them unpeeled! I had to explain this to them in my own glib blarney manner that I was taking advantage of the essential oil in the orange peel to get rid of toxins, as well as possible parasites in my digestive system.

Needless to say, I got all of them trying out unpeeled orange fruits, – washed before hand, of course, – and some of them making faces at the sharp taste of the orange rind and peel.

In fact, historically, many countries with a tropical and warm climate have made up a diet, which cools the system, and prevents problems of digestion. That is why the food here is predominantly vegetarian.

Time-Tested Tips

Here are some time-tested tips, which you may find interesting, to get rid of ailments.

If you drink water three hours before you have to have a meal, it is going to cool down the heat in your intestines and make it easier for you to digest food properly. Also, you are going to be surprised to note, that it is going to be easier for you to digest, a number of hot spices and even rich foods.

That means if you drink water beforehand without eating anything else in between, and eating a meal three hours later, you may find your digestion improving tremendously.

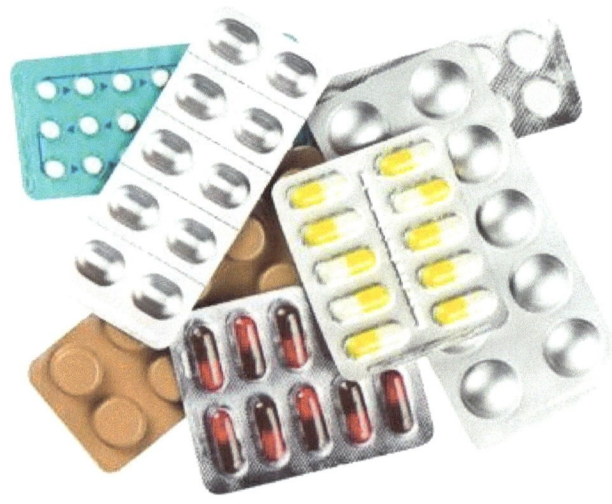

Do you think that these are responsible for keeping you healthy?

The ancients believed that medicines were not there to cure ailments. They were just there to relieve the symptoms and after that, it was the job of the wise people well versed in herbal lore, and medicine to make sure that that disease did not occur again. That is why they advocated that the patient build up his energy again, after an illness by eating proper and nourishing food.

Unfortunately today, we have got so used to popping pills that we do not allow the body to cure itself or heal itself, naturally. Instead, we try shortcuts like antibiotics which not only gets rid of the infection but also gets rid of all the useful bacteria which would have helped cure our bodies faster. And that means, that we are going to be prey to other diseases. And that means we are going to take even more medicines to get rid of the diseases, which were caused by the side effects of the medicines we took for getting rid of one particular disease.

This is a really vicious circle and a catch-22 situation, wouldn't you think.

So far as it is possible, keep away from prescribed drugs and medicines. You may see that most of them have nasty side effects, which your doctor is going to tell you is due to medicines. He has prescribed them to you. After six months, he is going to prescribe even more medicines to get rid of the temporarily cured disease, which was put into abeyance by the use of antibiotics.

So what happens after six months? You are still ill.

These natural tips can help you keep healthy, in these particular diseases situation, and they are time-tested.

Anybody suffering from fever, especially malaria and chronic fever should be given lots of milk, oranges, citrus fruits, and sugarcane juice. When he recovers from the fever, he should be given tapioca pudding, soup of beans and lentils, onion soup, and porridge. Do not give him solid things to eat.

Here is a delicious nourishing tomato soup for when he is better and wants to eat more solid proteinaceous things.

For this you need **25 g of butter, one bay leaf, three pieces of cinnamon crushed with five pieces of cardamoms - crushed, 5 g of roasted cumin seeds - ground, 25 g of garlic – 3/4 cloves – crushed, five crushed peppercorns, 750 g of tomatoes - chopped into bite-size pieces and deseeded, 25 g of rock salt, salt and pepper to taste.**

Put the butter in the saucepan and allow to heat. Now put the bay leaf, cinnamon, and other spices, cloves of garlic, pepper, salt, and rock salt in this mixture, and roast it gently.

Put the tomatoes in this mixture, and allow to cook for the next 45 minutes on low heat.

Garnish with some butter, parsley leaves, black salt and some roasted cumin seeds, ground well. Serve hot.

I love this in the winter. This is a healthy, nourishing, and one can always say a grateful drink, especially when you have come in from the cold. I love it with hot buttered toast as a snack, or even as dinner when I am too lazy to cook something fresh. I make this, in large quantities and put it in the fridge, and take out just the amount needed, nevertheless, finishing it up, before the week is over. Because what is fresh is delicious, what needs to be reheated may turn out to be really monotonous.

If you are suffering from tonsils, gargle with hot water in which you have put a little bit of powdered alum and salt. You can also gargle with hot water in which you have boiled tea leaves. Filter and gargle.

Diarrhea

If you are suffering from diarrhea, eat yogurt, rice, buttermilk, a ripe banana – one, because that is going to cause constipation, two bananas open up your system! – and unpeeled apples.

You may also want to eat Kedgeree which is a dish of rice and lentils. Good for Convalescents, and extra good for anybody who is looking for a light meal.

Traditional Khichri

[Literally mung dal hotch potch. In Britain, this dish is eaten for breakfast, with fish added and is called kedgeree.]

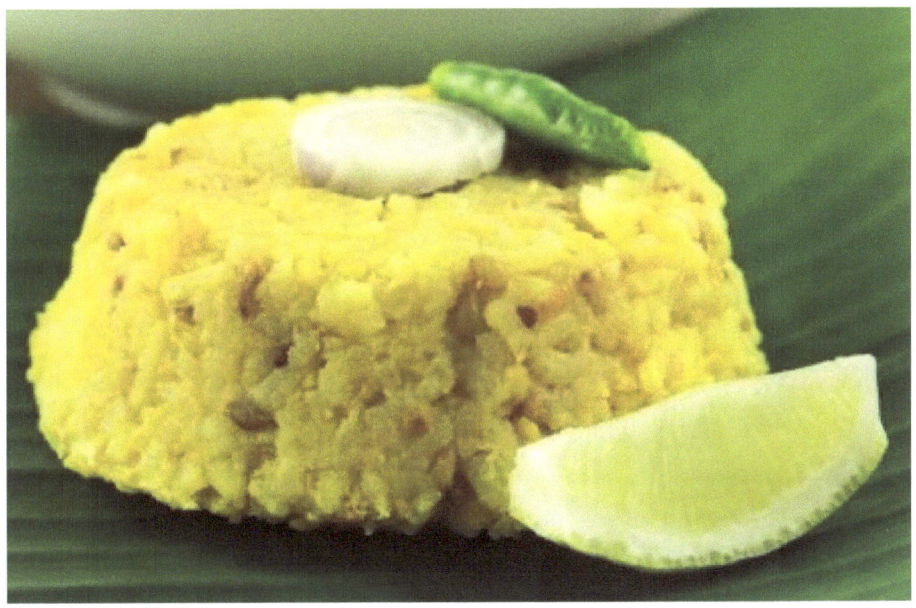

1/2 Cup - Yellow or green Moong Dal

1 Cup Basmati Rice

To Taste - Salt

5-6 Cups - Water

For Tadka/seasoning

2 Tsp - Ghee/Oil

3-4 - Green Chili

A Pinch - Asafoetida/Hing

1 tsp - Cumin Seeds/Jeera

2 tsp - Minced Garlic

Clean the rice as well as the mung and then soak it for 15 minutes. Add three cups water to the rice and the dal and allow to cook until the water is absorbed.

If you have a pressure cooker, allow it to 'whistle" thrice. That means that this is going to be cooked into porridge consistency.

It takes a while for green mung to be cooked, so we are going to remove it from the heat and mash it up along with the rice with a spoon and a little bit of oil/ghee – clarified butter. Then put it on the boil again with one more cup water. This quantity is going to depend on how watery or how thick you want your porridge to be.

If you are going to be using it as comfort food, you can do the tempering. If you are going to be using it as food for invalids, just add rock salt, pepper and a little bit of lemon juice sprinkled on top, and give it to your patient with a bowl of yogurt. This is easy to digest. Do not eat it with pickles, if you are suffering from dysentery/diarrhea, and want to cure it. After you have been cured, you can eat it with anything!

Tempering is what is going to give that extra touch of yumminess to this Khichdi.

Mix the garlic with the cumin seeds and chop the chilies. Heat the oil in your frying pan, add garlic and asafetida, and fry until it is a Golden brown. Now add the chilies and fry until you hear the crackle of the cumin.

This tempering is poured straight over the khichadi and mixed. It is then served hot with yogurt, pickles, and your favorite salads. Enjoy, because this is made of the most easily digested foods.

There is another traditional way in which you can get rid of diarrhea. Just rub some nutmeg in some water until you have a brown paste. Put this in a glass of water, and allow the patient to drink it, three times a day. This is going to stop the diarrhea.

Jaundice

People suffering from jaundice can benefit by drinking lots of fresh sugarcane juice, grape juice, and eating fresh green leafy vegetables, along with drinking fresh fruit and vegetable juices.

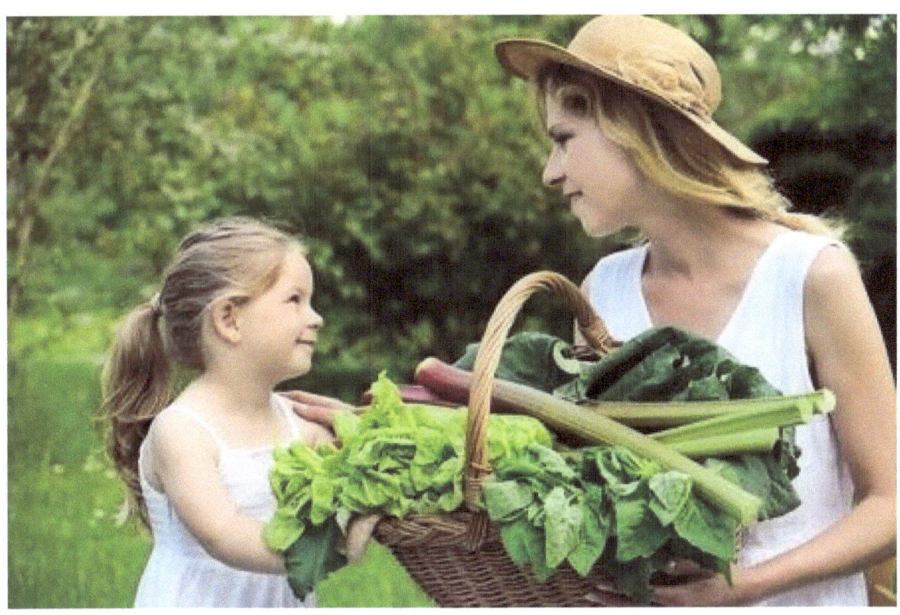

Lots of greens means a healthy life and a healthy lifestyle!

Eczema

People suffering from eczema, skin ailments, boils, or hives, should stop eating fried foods. They should not drink tea. They should start eating more spinach, reddish leaves, tomatoes, onions, carrots, and papayas. Apply a mixture of turpentine oil and juice from a couple of cloves of garlic on the affected areas until this disappears. It is going to take anywhere between a week to 15 days depending on the seriousness of the case.

People suffering from gout should not eat spinach, bananas, and potatoes in the same way, people suffering from diabetes should not eat bananas, and sweet food items.

People suffering from ulcers should not eat oranges, lemons, and sour fruits, instead they should pep up their intake of milk with honey and milk with turmeric. For milk with turmeric, you need to put half a teaspoonful of turmeric powder, into freshly boiled milk, cooling down, in which you have put a teaspoonful of honey. Drink this down. This is going to help heal your ulcer really fast. It is also going to get rid of any infection in your body, including muscular sprains, aches, and other possible problems in your muscles and tissues.

Cough and cold

If you suffer from persistent cough and cold, you may want to stop drinking milk and eating milk products. This includes buttermilk, ice cream, cheese, and other delicious dairy products. Also, try to avoid fried foods of any sort, including chips, or any sort of pride comfort food, which you want to eat just because you are feeling low due to a cold.

Chickenpox

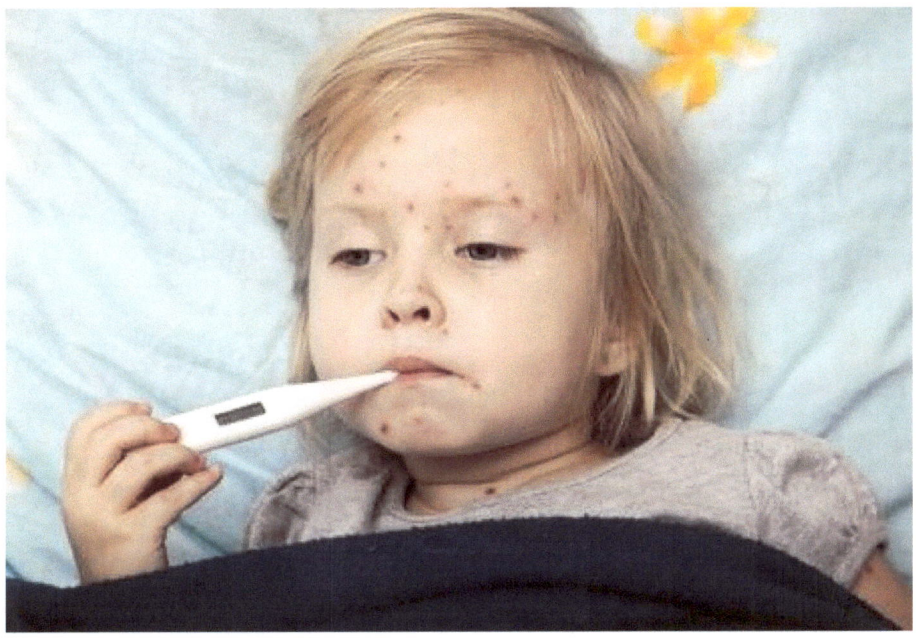

This is one suffering from chickenpox should be fed lots of milk, grapes, pomegranates, citrus fruits like oranges, and other juicy fruits as much as she wants to eat and drink. This is going to help heal her faster.

Sciatica

People suffering from sciatica find themselves nearly immobilized with the sharp pang of pain going through their system all of a sudden. Especially in the lower back.

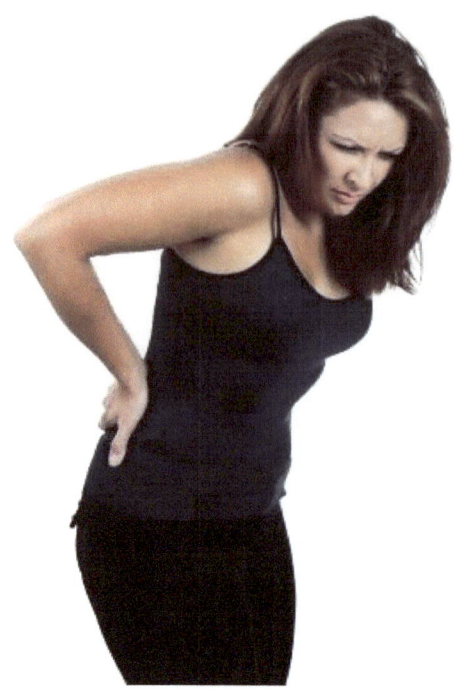

If you are suffering from sciatica, stop eating yogurt, bananas, rice, radishes, potatoes, and sour foods like pickles, tomatoes, and even some sour sauces.

Healthy Vegetarian Dishes

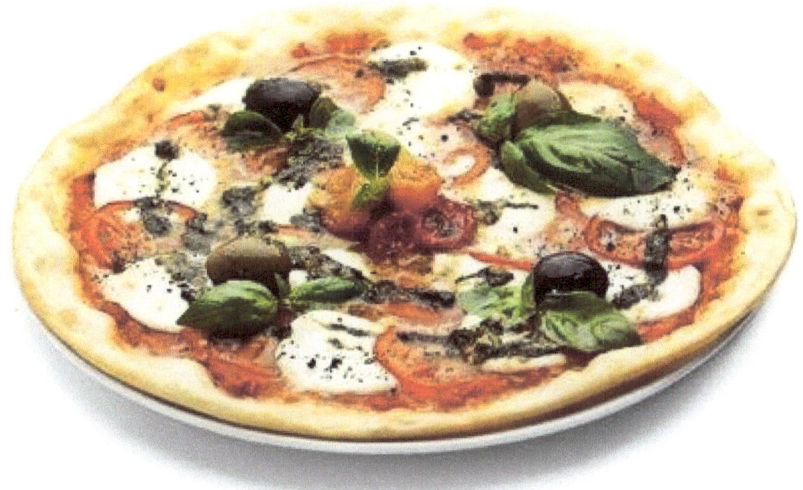

Traditional Pizza

It takes 25 minutes for you to make this pizza and 10 minutes to cook it. Two people can dine well off it, but when I make it, it satisfies me and everybody else look to other means.

For the pizza base, you are going to need 300 g of whole-wheat bread flour, 1 teaspoon instant yeast, 1 teaspoon salt, 200 mL of hot water, 1 tablespoon full of olive oil with a little bit of extra for basting on the top.

For the tomato sauce, you are going to need hundred milligrams of pizza sauce – [recipe given further on], some leaves of basin, one clove of garlic minced, salt-and-pepper, according to taste.

For the topping you need 125 g of pizza cheese or mozzarella cheese, sliced, a little bit of Parmesan cheese just for a change of taste – I like cheddar – two tomatoes, four cherry tomatoes, cut into wedges or slices, a little bit of olive oil for sprinkling on the top.

Garnishing with basil leaves. You may also want to garnish with olives, as done traditionally.

Put the flour in a large bowl, and add the pepper and the salt as well as the yeast to it. Now make a hollow in the middle of the flour and add 200 mL hot water and the olive oil. Mix well with a wooden spatula.

Now flour a flat surface and knead the flour upon it, until you have dough which is not too stiff. Cover this dough with a moist tea towel, and allow to ferment for about two hours. However, if you are making a pizza without any crust, you do not need to ferment it.

Mix the pizza sauce, basil leaves, and the garlic together in a bowl. Add salt-and-pepper, according to your taste. Allow this mixture to remain at room temperature, while the pizza base is fermenting on its own.

If you allowed the flour to ferment, you will have to knock it back, which means kneading it yet once again. Now cut the dough into two equal parts. Each part is going to be rolled with a rolling pin on a floured surface. Make a rolled out circle, 25 cm in diameter. Make sure that it is thin, because when you are going to make it, it is going to swell up like a normal pizza.

Do the same for the second part also. Sprinkle some flour on some baking sheets, and place it ready for baking. Heat the oven to 240°C (450°F). Put an extra baking tray, upside down on the topmost shelf of your oven or you can put another baking sheet, there.

Put these items in layers on your pizza base. The lower most layer is going to be made up of your pizza sauce and basil leaf mixture. After that, you are going to put a layer of tomatoes on. Sprinkle the mozerella and Parmesan on top of the tomato layer. Cover with olive oil and any other herbal salt if you like.

Allow one pizza base along with topping to bake on the already heated sheet/upturned portion of the baking tray, and allow to bake for 8 to 10 minutes. Serve garnished with basil leaves, and a sprinkling of olive oil.

Here are some tips, which you may want to utilize, when you are making your pizza for the first time. What happens if the dough is really wet and sticky? Just add some fresh flour and allow the dry flour to counteract the power of all that water.

What happens when you find it difficult to roll out the fresh dough? Leave it for another 10 minutes. After that, try to roll it out again. Remember that this particular dough is going to take more effort to roll out, than what is taken when you roll out pastry dough.

What if the base has not cooked properly. You need to put the pizza on an already heated sheet or baking tray. If that has been done beforehand, your pizza base will never be on cooked. Also, the base should not be really really thick, as is offered by a number of pizza brands calling it a double pizza. Also make sure that you do not overloaded with topping, because that could possibly prevent the pizza base from cooking.

So if you find that the topping has been baked, first, before the pizza base, cover it with a foil, and allow to cook for five minutes more.

Traditional Pizza sauce –Passata sauce

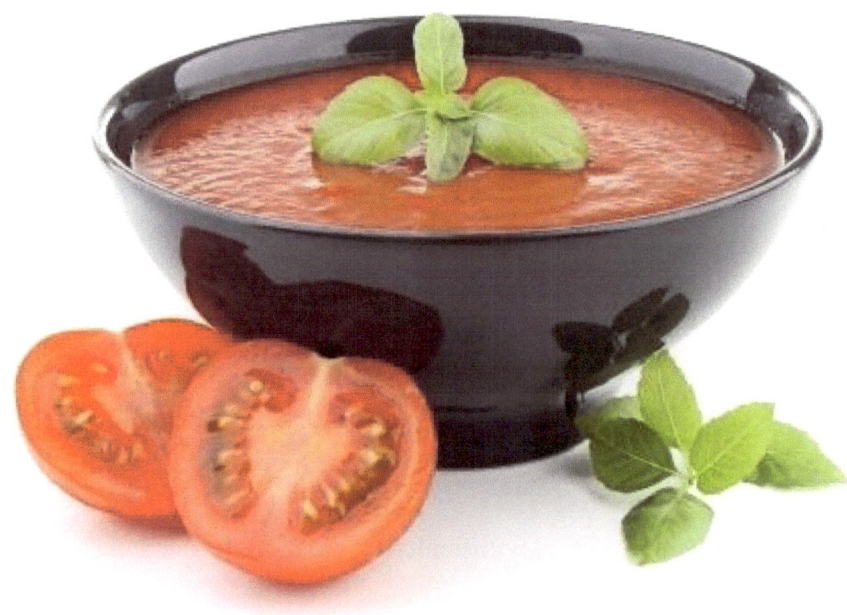

Apart from soups, tomatoes are delicious and an important part of pizza sauces as Passata sauces.

This traditional recipe calls for plenty of tomatoes along with herbs. For this you are going to need **10 ripe tomatoes - pulped and deseeded, 1 tablespoon full of Worcestershire sauce, three bulbs of garlic - crushed and roasted, 2 tablespoons full of olive oil, one teaspoonful of sugar, salt** and pepper to taste, half a teaspoonful of paprika or chili powder, 1 tablespoon full of Oregano, a mixture of any of your favorite herbs – when I am making passata I take hefty pinches of all my favorite herbs, including basil, thyme, marjoram, parsley, and anything else available in my kitchen cupboard at that time, – and just a little bit of cream.

Put the olive oil into your frying pan, and add the tomatoes. Add the garlic, roasting them makes it even tastier, the Worcestershire sauce and the sugar. Do the seasoning with pepper and salt.

Now allowed to cook, while mashing the tomatoes so that they have a smooth consistency, and simmer. Strain this in another bowl to get rid of the lumpy material and allow to cook for another seven minutes on simmer speed. You can mash the lumpy material again, and mix it in the simmering sauce.

This is your pizza sauce, which you can refrigerate and use as a base topping on your pizza base, whenever you want.

Spinach With Cream

Spinach cooked with herbs and spices, and served with cream is a really delicious and healthy dish.

Preparation time 20 minutes, cooking time 15 minutes serving four really hungry people.

For this you need 500 g of well washed spinach, 200 g of cottage cheese, half a teaspoon each of ground cumin seeds, ground fenugreek, turmeric powder, coriander powder, 2 tablespoons full of chopped walnuts, salt to taste. Three onions - chopped up fine, one teaspoonful of

chopped ginger, three cloves of garlic, chopped fine, 20 mL yogurt, and Oil for frying.

Blanch the spinach by putting it in boiling hot water. After that, take it out and put it in cold water for two minutes. Blend it well until you have a spinach purée.

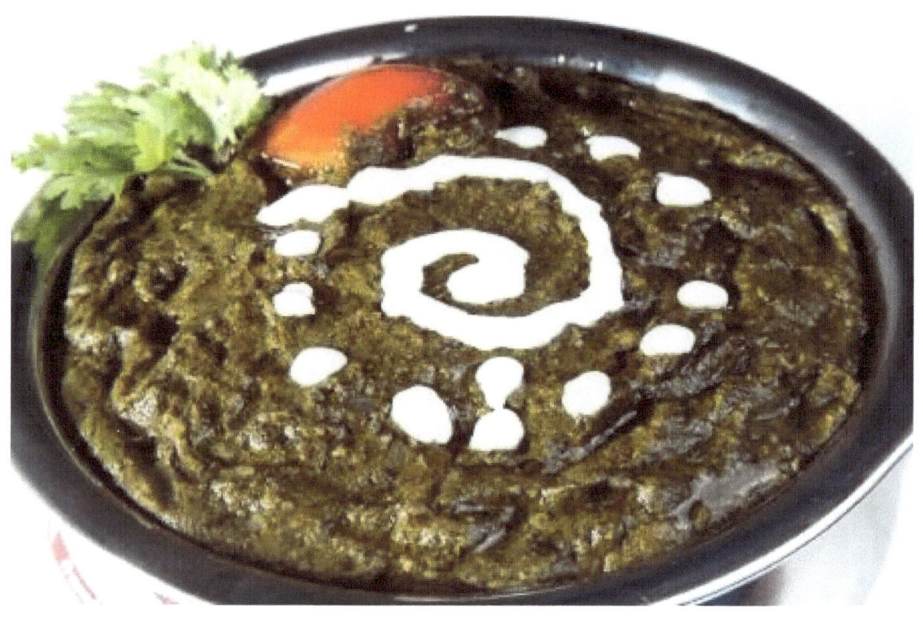

Grate the cottage cheese. Now add the walnuts, spices, and salt. Mix this up by kneading it like a Dough. Make small cottage cheese balls out of this mixture. Heat the oil in the frying pan and fry these balls in it until they are golden brown. Remove, drain and allow to cool.

Now add 10 mL of oil in a Wok. Put the fenugreek seeds in the hot oil, and the onion. Allow to fry until golden brown. After that, add the ginger and the garlic and continue frying until all of them are a rich golden brown.

Now add some cumin powder to this mixture, and coriander powder as well as the turmeric. Mix well.

Now put the spinach purée in this mixture and allow to cook on a medium heat until bubbling. Whip the yogurt and add salt to taste. Add the yogurt to this mixture, and allow to cook.

Now add the fried cottage cheese balls, stir once and remove from fire.

Garnish with coriander leaves and with cream. Serve piping hot.

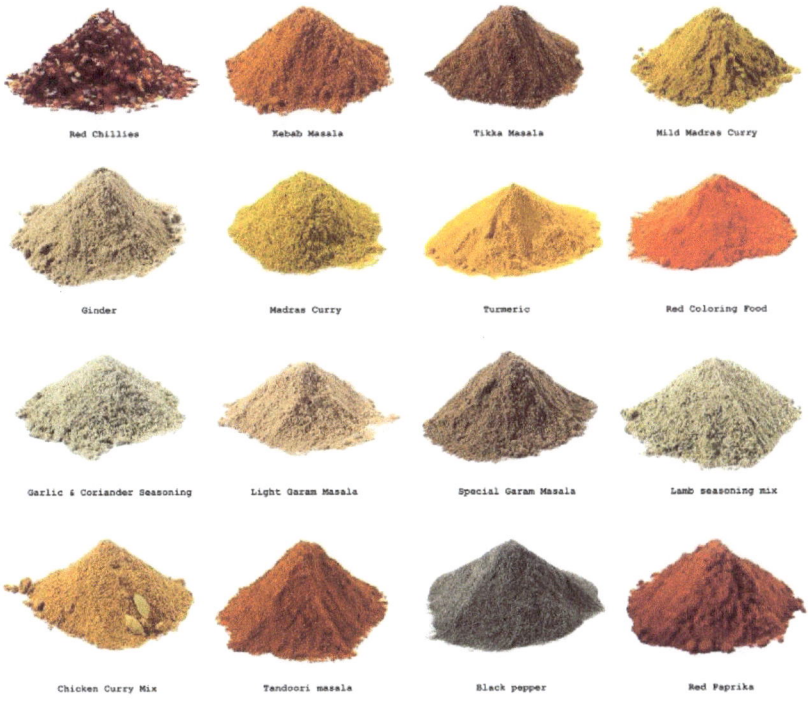

These are some of the spices, which are commonly used to make even the most bland of meals and dishes, delicious.

Conclusion

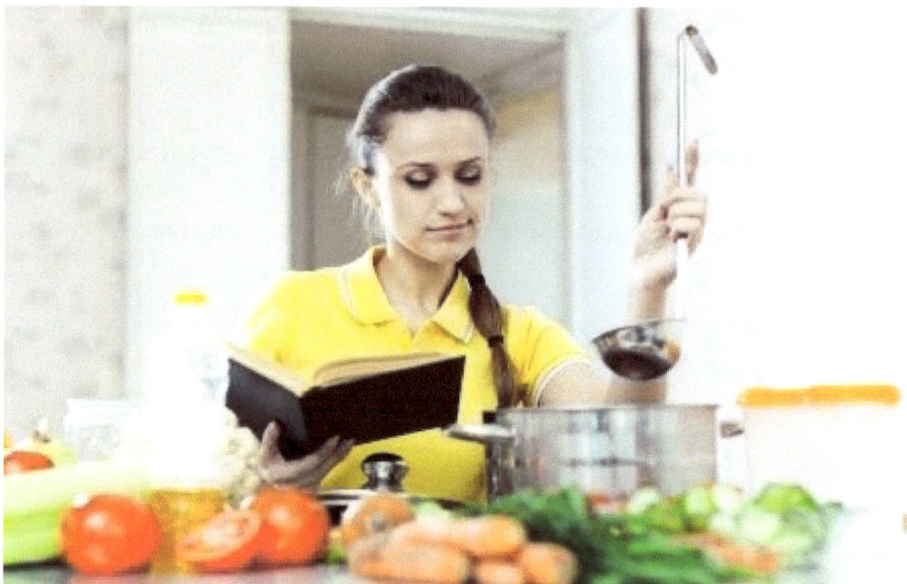

This book is for all of those people who just cannot resist biting into a juicy steak or filet mignon or a hamburger with a delicious juicy beef burger. I was hundred percent omnivorous, with the balance shifting towards the carnivorous, and becoming an herbivore was too much of a lifestyle change for me.

Until I had to live in a place, where culturally, religiously, and traditionally, nobody ate meat. Those six years were the healthiest years of my life, until of course I came back into the mainstream Metropolitan lifestyle, and changed my eating habits accordingly.

So remember, if you cannot stop eating all that meat right at once – and I am not telling you to do so, even though I am trying to be a herbivore, I retrogressive, whenever I smell barbecued pork chops, especially those made by my father, marinated in herbs, garlic, yogurt, turmeric, vodka, and anything else of which you could think and allowed to steep for 48 hours – I would dare a hermit to pass this by…, Try reducing your intake of meat.

So when you eat meat, three times a day, start eating it twice a day. After two months, get to once a day. Within six months, you will have forgotten how to the craving for sausages, bacon, hamburger, and other juicy meat preparations made you wake up at night saying, where is my fryer, I am hungry![1]

So live healthy, Live Long and Prosper!

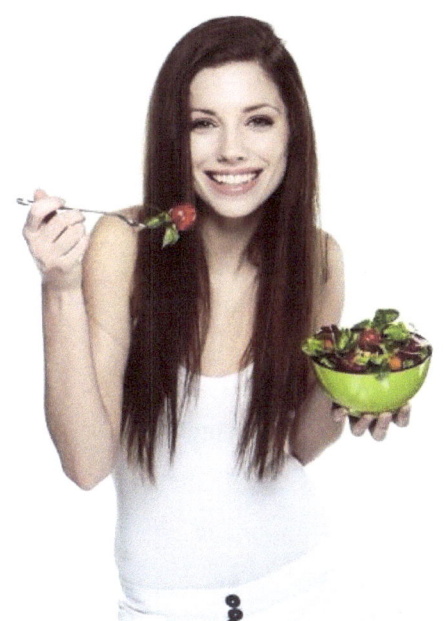

---

[1] Been there, done that, often, and often, especially with bacon butties and fried eggs at midnight, with lots of butter and cheese. This fare is conducive to insomnia, but what a way to go! Naturally, the next morning I have to run 1 extra mile in order to stay fit.

Author Bio

Dueep Jyot Singh is a Management and IT Professional who managed to gather Postgraduate qualifications in Management and English and Degrees in Science, French and Education while pursuing different enjoyable career options like being an hospital administrator, IT,SEO and HRD Database Manager/ trainer, movie , radio and TV scriptwriter, theatre artiste and public speaker, lecturer in French, Marketing and Advertising, ex-Editor of Hearts On Fire (now known as Solstice) Books Missouri USA, advice columnist and cartoonist, publisher and Aviation School trainer, ex-moderator on Medico.in, banker, student councilor ,travelogue writer … among other things!

One fine morning, she decided that she had enough of killing herself by Degrees and went back to her first love—writing. It's more enjoyable! She already has 48 published academic and 14 fiction- in- different- genre books under her belt.

When she is not designing websites or making Graphic design illustrations for clients , she is browsing through old bookshops hunting for treasures, of which she has an enviable collection – including R.L. Stevenson, O.Henry, Dornford Yates, Maurice Walsh, De Maupassant, Victor Hugo, Sapper, C.N. Williamson, "Bartimeus" and the crown of her collection- Dickens "The Old Curiosity Shop," and "Martin Chuzzlewit" and so on… Just call her "Renaissance Woman" - collecting herbal remedies, acting like Universal Helping Hand/Agony Aunt, or escaping to her dear mountains for a bit of exploring, collecting herbs and plants, and trekking.

Check out some of the other JD-Biz Publishing books

Gardening Series on Amazon

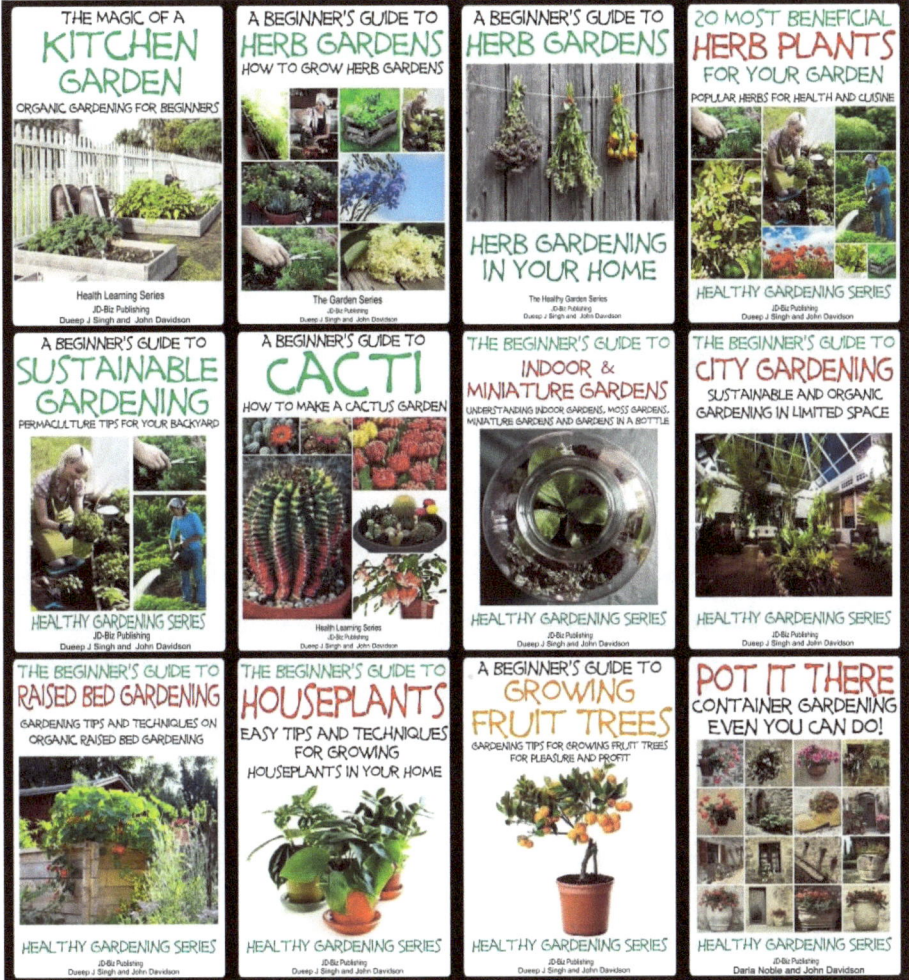

Download Free Books!

http://MendonCottageBooks.com

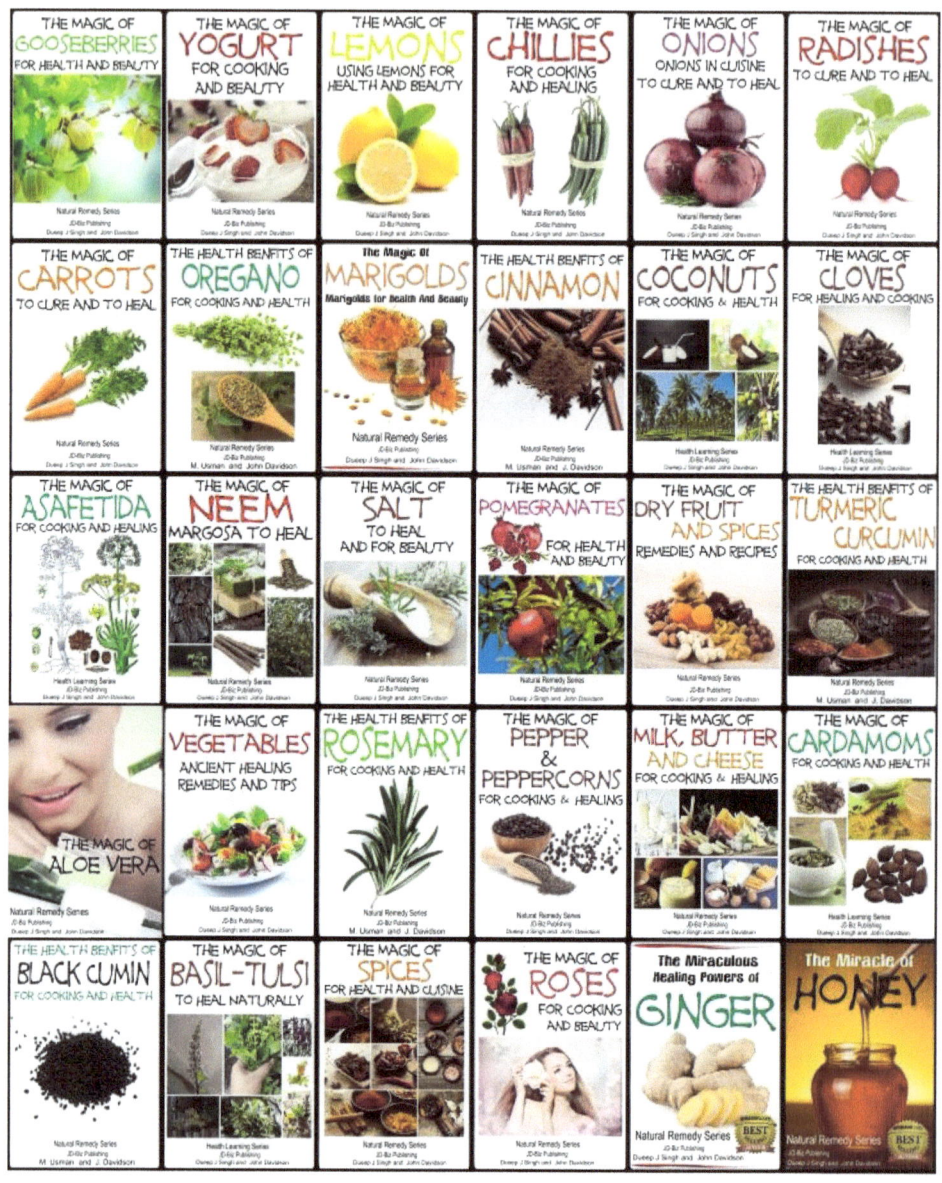

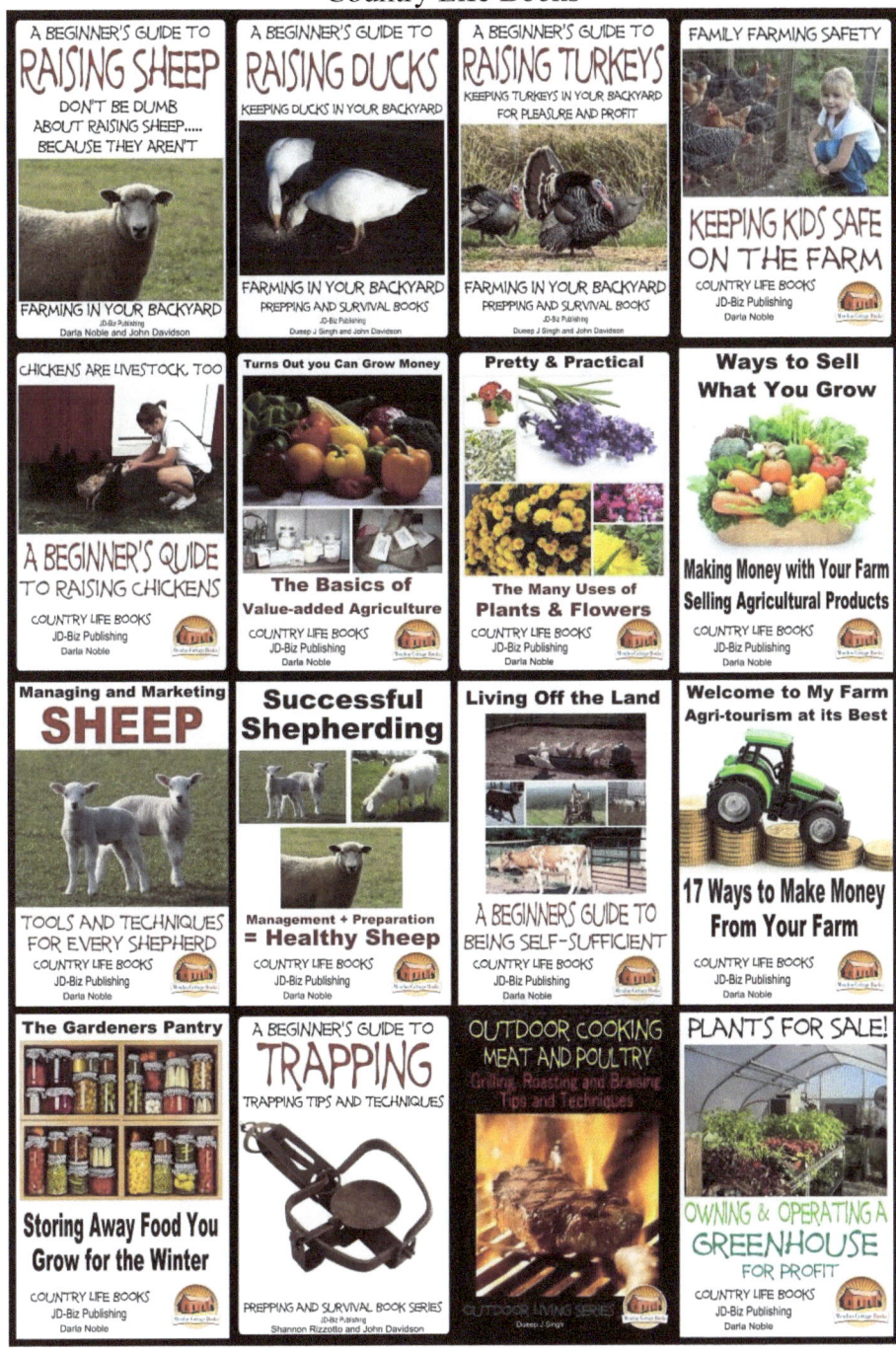

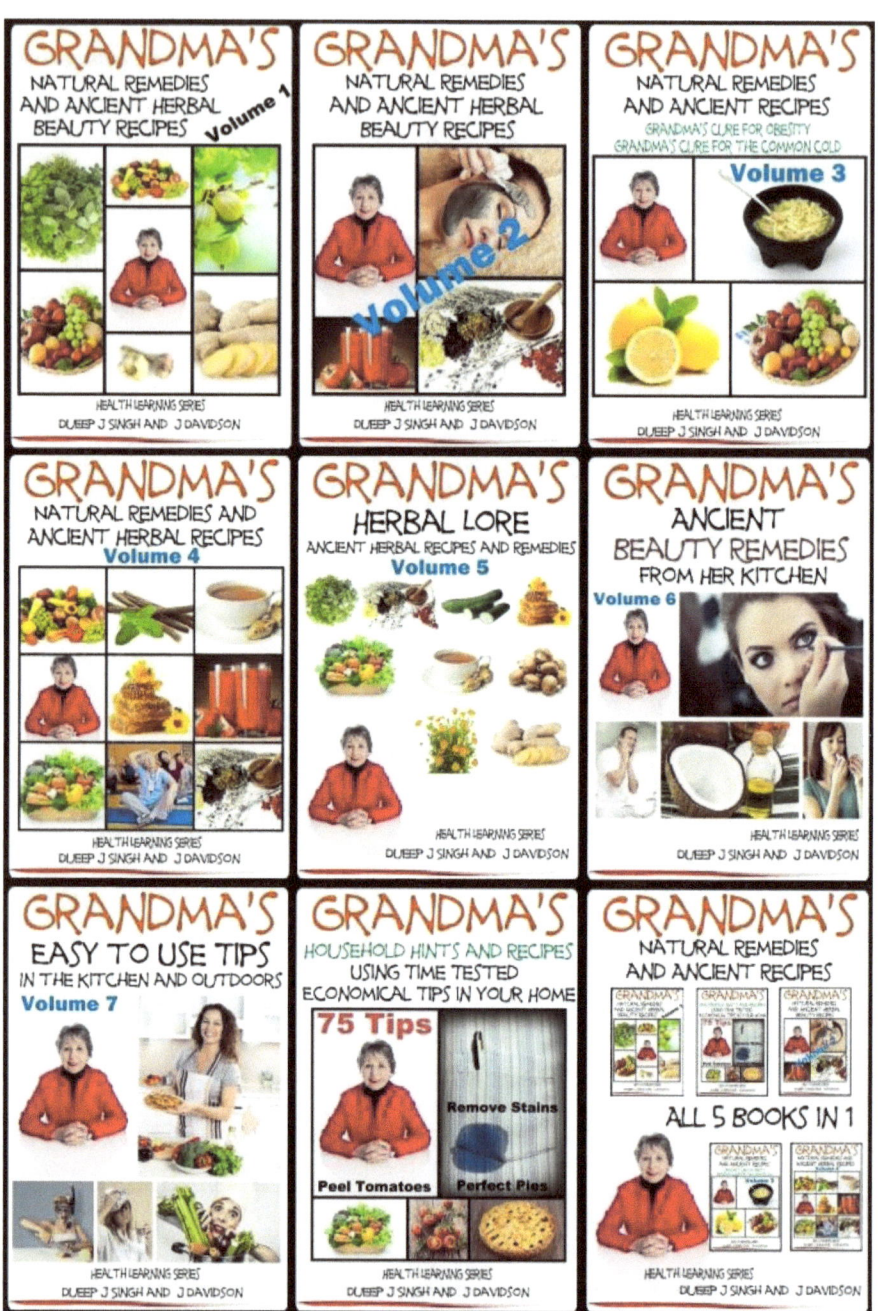

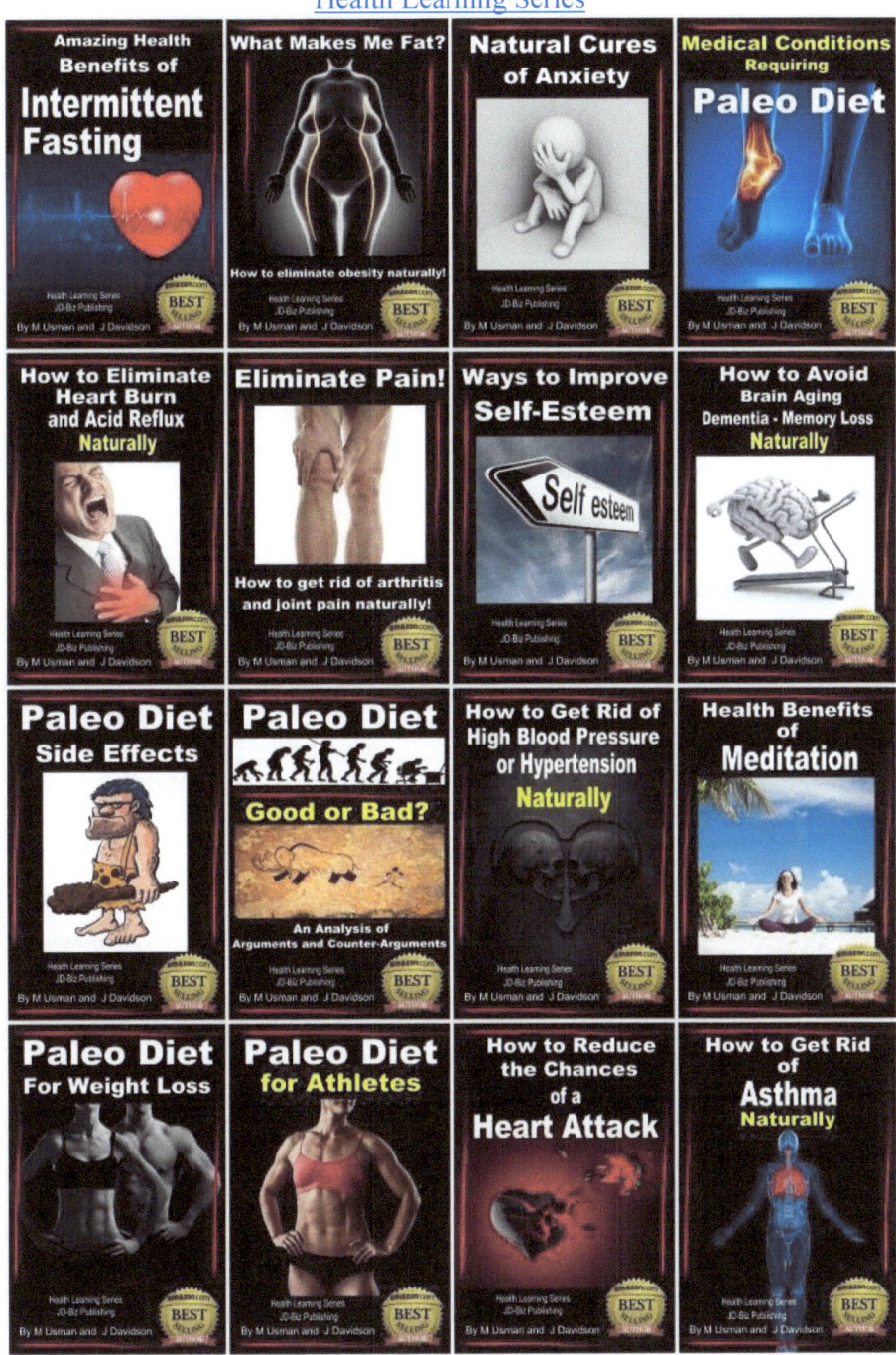

Amazing Animal Book Series

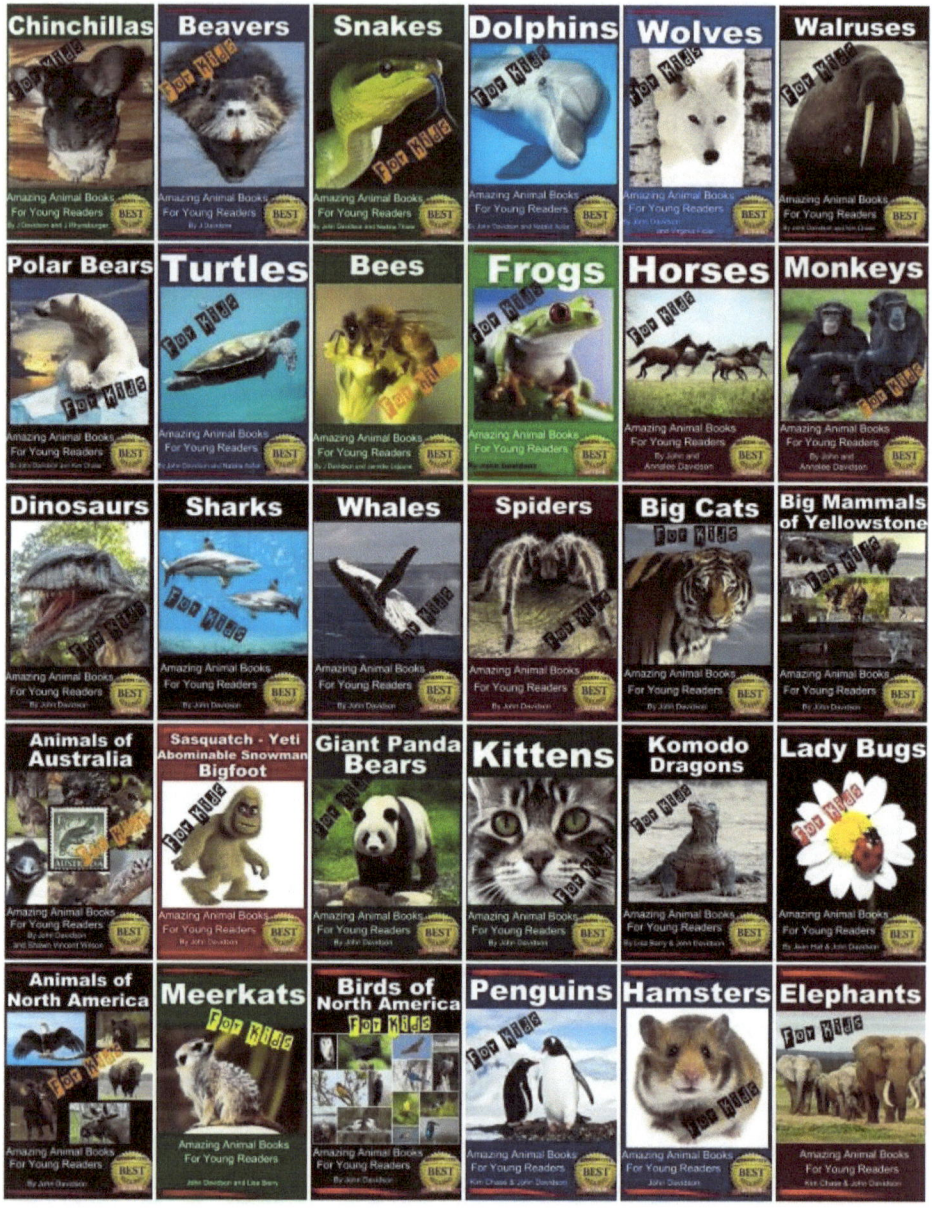

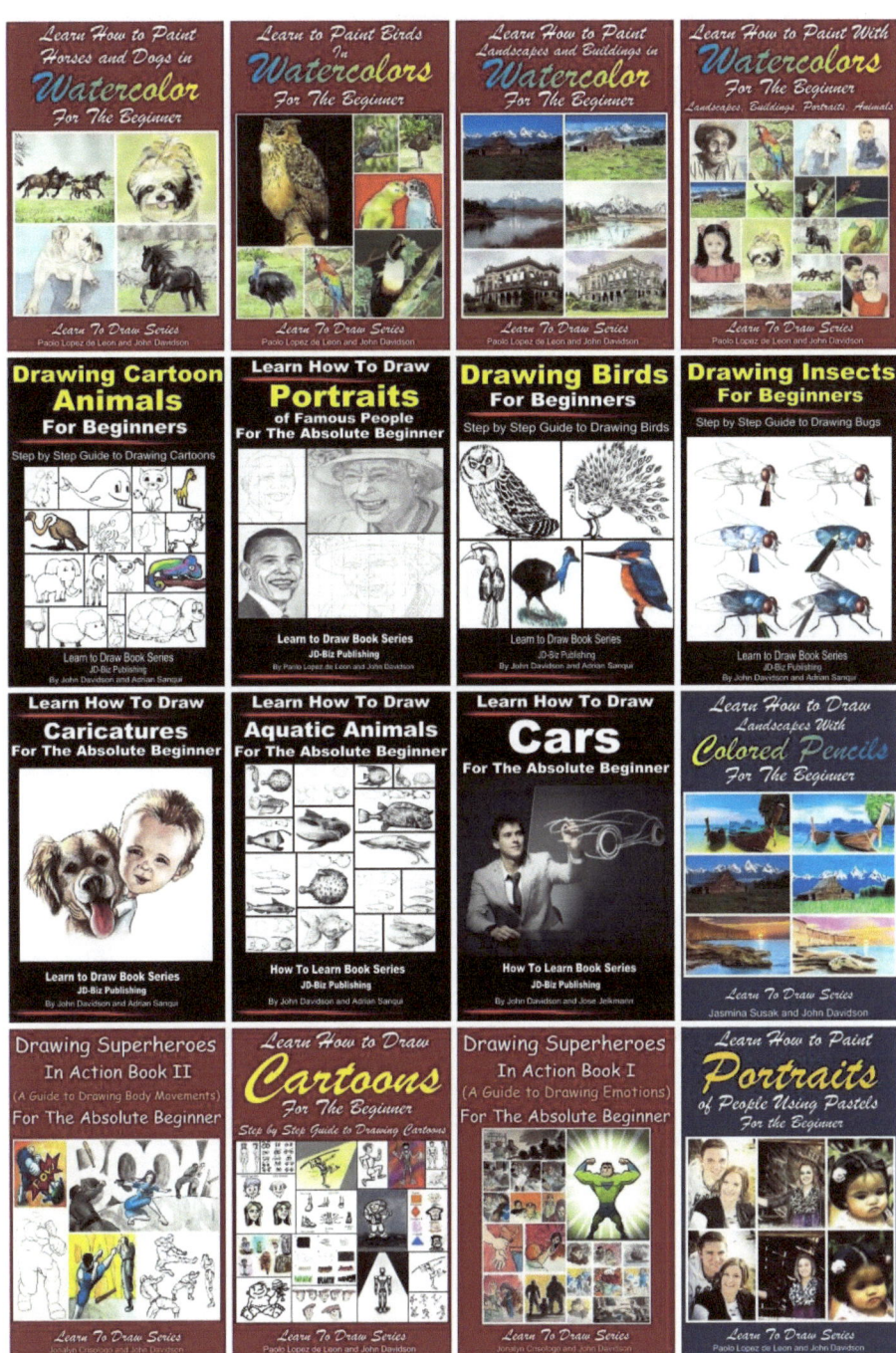

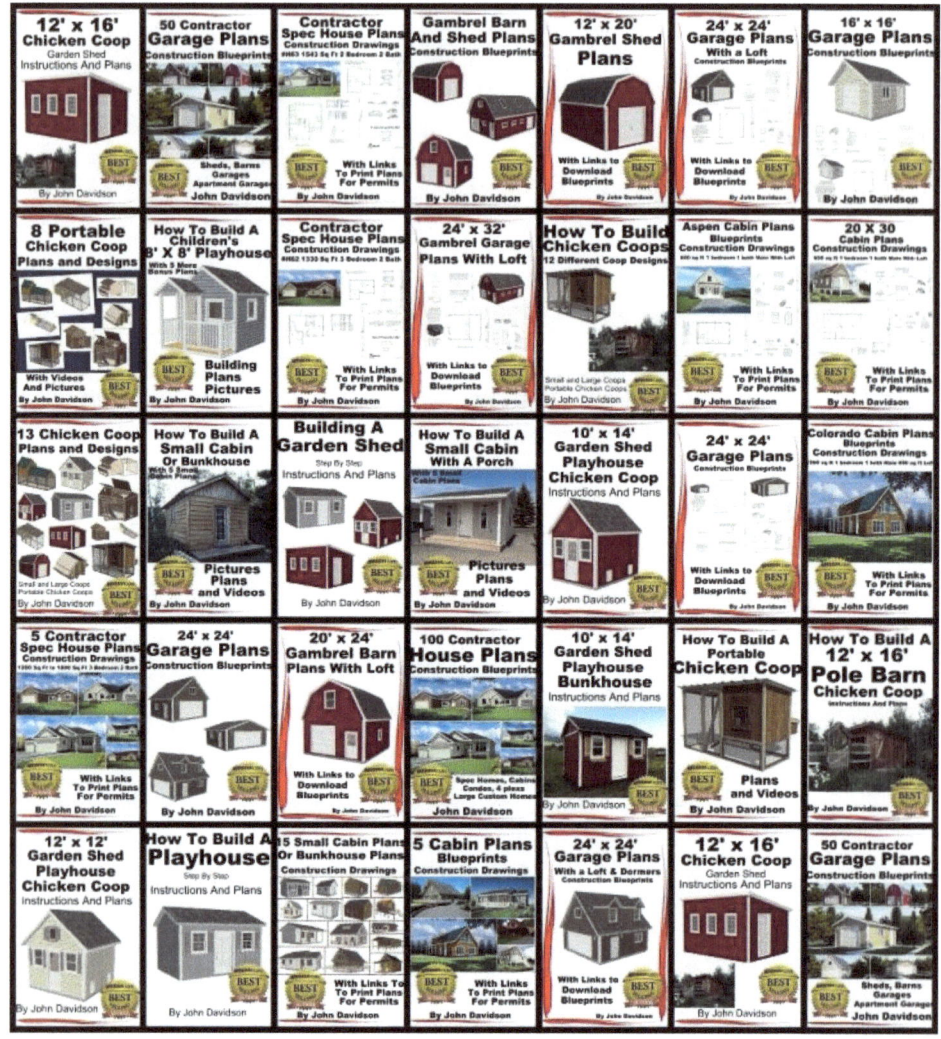

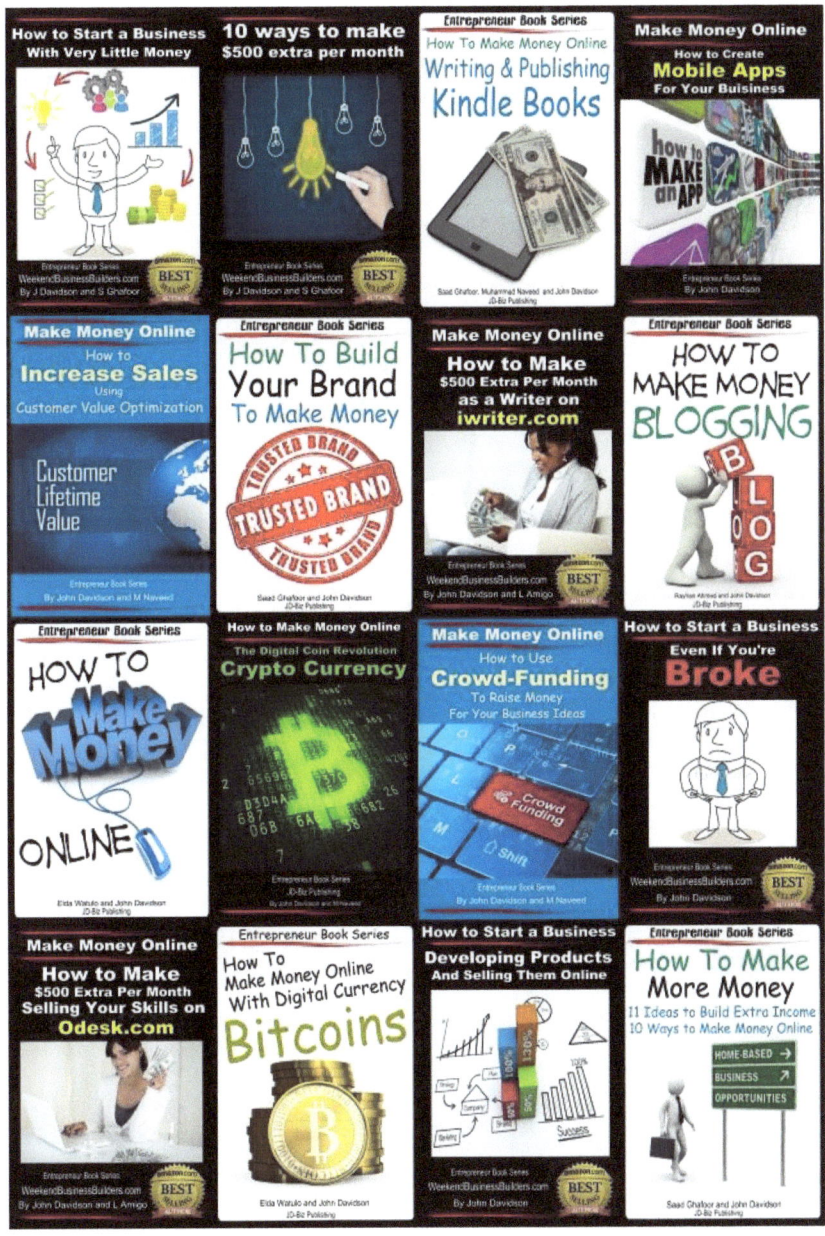

Our books are available at

1. Amazon.com

2. Barnes and Noble

3. Itunes

4. Kobo

5. Smashwords

6. Google Play Books

Download Free Books!

http://MendonCottageBooks.com

Publisher

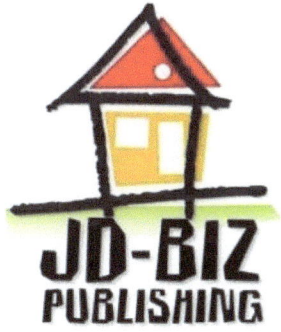

JD-Biz Corp

P O Box 374

Mendon, Utah 84325

http://www.jd-biz.com/

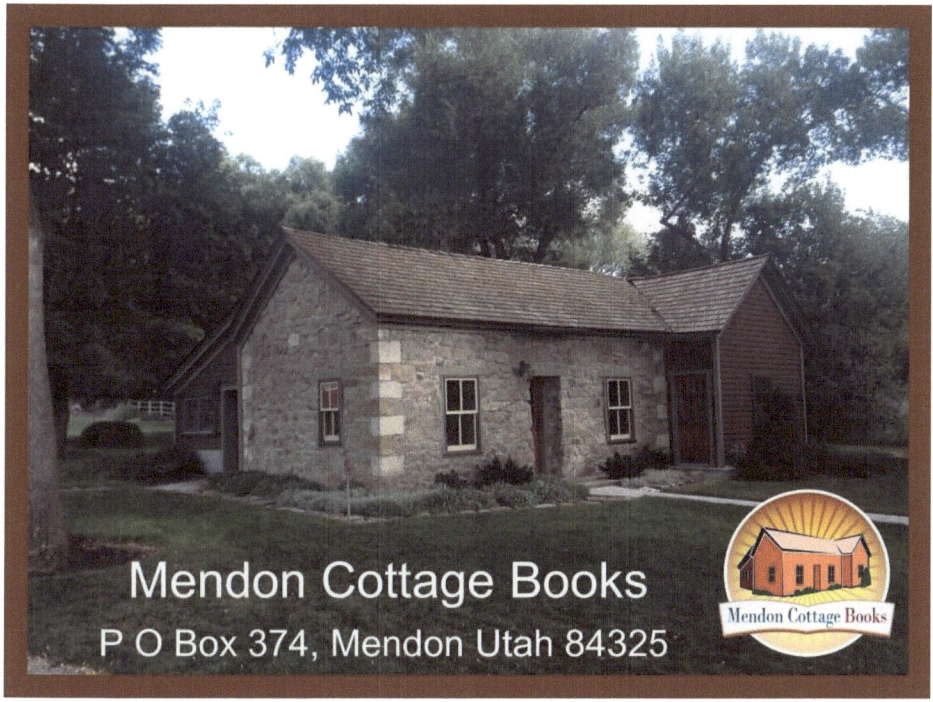

www.ingramcontent.com/pod-product-compliance
Lightning Source LLC
Chambersburg PA
CBHW050821290526
45792CB00001B/208